WEIGHT LOSS BY GINA

WINTER 2022 PROGRAM

Posts and Guidelines

ISBN: 9798786039055

We are committed to making weight loss as easy as possible. In doing so, we have put together this booklet containing the instructional information which will be posted in the Winter 2022 Group week to week. Please keep in mind this booklet does NOT contain all of the information and posts, so you will still need to check into the Group day to day to review any newly added information and to watch the videos that go along with these posts.

At the end of this document, you will also find some tracking sheets that you can use to track your progress. The tracking sheets will help you pick up on patterns of behaviour and how your body is responding to the changes you are making day to day.

I also want to acknowledge and thank Andrea Mut, Anna Blachuta, Krystyna Recoskie, and Kim Turnbull for contributing content that is included in this booklet. Special thanks also goes out to Terry-Ann Pighin, Kim Johnstone for their help in bringing it all together, and Chrissy Hobbs from Indie Publishing Group, who helped with all the editing and formatting. Thank you so much for all your efforts and this booklet wouldn't be possible without your help.

Disclaimer: These documents do not contain medical/health advice. The information is provided for general informational and educational purposes only and is not a substitute for professional advice. Please speak to your healthcare provider if you have any concerns before starting and/or during the Program.

CONTENTS

WELCOME TO GINA'S WINTER 2022 WEIGHT LOSS PROGRAM

LET'S GET STARTED WITH PREP WEEK!

If you are new to the Program, Prep Week is all about reviewing the basics, like the Food Plan you are to follow, how the program works, as well as gather anything you might need and ask any questions you have. It's not about being perfect, it's about understanding the process and setting yourself up for success.

If you are a returning member, Prep Week is all about getting back at it and setting yourself up for success as you continue your weight loss journey on the road to finally & forever.

WHAT IS THE LIVY METHOD:

- The Livy Method is about losing weight in a way that is healthy for the body and mind so weight loss is easier to maintain.

- The approach is to systematically lower your setpoint by addressing weight loss from a variety of different angles, physically and mentally, week to week. Your setpoint is the weight your body is used to functioning at - also known as homeostasis - where all the regulatory systems in your body work together to maintain balance for the purpose of helping the body survive and work at its most optimal level.

- There is a basic Food Plan you will need to follow where each week will have a different focus, so keep in mind what you eat and when you eat will change and evolve week to week.

HOW THE PROGRAM WORKS:

- The Program is broken down into a step-by-step process (The Livy Method) designed to systematically address why your body is feeling a need to store fat and help it focus on fat loss, so you can sustainably lose as much weight as you can in the time frame we have.

- What you eat and when you eat will change week to week as The Program progresses. Each week will have a different focus, although the kinds of foods you eat will stay the same (see Grocery List).

- The best way to approach the program is to check into the Facebook Group each day to watch the Daily Check in Video as well as any other added support videos/posts which will give a more detailed explanation of any changes you are advised to implement.

- The Facebook Support Group is also where you are to ask any questions if you have them.

- Each day, we will post a question board where you can ask any questions you have.

- Questions will be answered by Gina and her team of Vibe Ambassadors, as well as many previous group members. Group members' answers will always be confirmed by a member of our team.

- Gina will be going Live Monday Friday in the Group at 9 -10AM, Saturday at 10 -11AM & Monday to Thursday at 78PM, all times in EST.

- The Live segments are not mandatory. All the info you need will be posted in the Group. The Live segments are saved in the GUIDES to be viewed later.

- This Program is very much designed to be followed day by day, week by week, for the full 12 weeks, regardless of how much weight you have to lose.

- With that said, it can also accommodate any time off or off day, and can be done on your own timeline.

- You can also use our new Livy Method app to journal and track your progress along the way.

DAILY CHECKLIST:

1. Read over the Weekly Basic Guidelines.

2. Check into the Support Group.

3. Watch the Daily Check In Video.

4. Ask your questions on the Daily Questions Post.

5. Watch/Review any additional Support Videos or Posts and click DONE to keep track of what you have read/watched.

6. Implement the changes you need to make.

7. Watch/participate in the Facebook Lives and ask questions. *Suggested but not Required*

It's pretty simple so don't overthink it. No need to weigh or measure your food or count any calories... just have faith in the Process.

We will be posting a lot of information over the next few days. Take your time to review and let us know if you have any questions. Also, be sure to check out the Table of Contents to check out all the topics we will be discussing week to week.

Please take time to head over to the Facebook Group and watch the quick video that accompanies this post.

3 WAYS TO GET YOUR QUESTIONS ASKED AND ANSWERED:

1. On the Daily Questions Post. This is pinned to the top of the Facebook Support Group page and is where you can ask any questions you have day to day.

2. Individual Posts. Each day we will be posting about a variety of different topics. Feel free to ask any questions you have about that topic on those posts.

3. If you choose, you can also participate and ask your questions by way of the Facebook Lives 9 am Mon Fri, 7pm Mon. - Thurs. and Saturday mornings at 10 am EST.

PLEASE NOTE:

*   Please avoid privately emailing your questions or sending DMs via social media, as our main focus while running the Group is to prioritize the questions being asked in it.

*   You will find the Program is laid out and designed to cover just about any and every question someone would have about the Program and process, so there is a lot to cover in the first few weeks.

*   Be sure to use the GUIDES to keep track of anything new being posted day to day and utilize the TOPICS section where you can also search specific topics that have been previously posted.

If you are feeling overwhelmed, trust we will be going over the info many times over and, as always, if you have questions let us know.

FAQS ABOUT THE PROGRAM

Here are some of our most popular questions asked about The Program:

1. **Is The Program low carb?**

   - No, although I do suggest taking out bread (except Ezekiel/Sprouted Grain and Ryvita/High Fiber crackers), all pasta, baked goods and obvious sugars. I have incorporated many nutrient rich and beneficial options for you to choose from.

2. **Do we have to weigh, measure, or count calories?**

   - No. Stick to the scheduled plan and portions will adjust on their own. Right now the key is to feel satisfied after each meal and snack. We will start to address portions in Weeks 3 and 4.

3. **What kind of results can I expect?**

   - Although the goal is to take as much weight off as quickly as possible, there is a process to it.

   - It is not unreasonable to expect upwards of a 60 lbs.+ loss for men and 40 lbs.+ loss for women, but that depends on the state of your body when you started, along with other variables. The average weight loss in our Fall 2021 group, based on a survey that was filled out by 4000 members, was 13.1 lbs. and the highest amount lost was 55 lbs.

   - Remember that this is not a quick fix program and it is meant to be followed day by day for the entire 12 weeks, regardless of how quickly you reach your goal.

   - Even if you have more weight to lose than possible in the time frame we have, the goal is to lose as much as possible and be well on your way to losing the rest once you complete the 12 weeks.

   - Everyone's body will respond differently and at different rates, so please be mindful not to rush the process or compare what is happening with you to what is happening with someone else.

4. **What can I expect in the first week?**

   - In the first week you may notice an increase in energy, a decrease in bloating, and more intense hunger signals. You may also experience a natural decrease in portion sizes and more pronounced "full" signals from the body.

   - Some of you will start dropping weight right away, while others may go into "repair and rebuild mode" in which case you might not see the scale move right away, but hang in there because it will…both are equally ideal.

   - As your body goes into weight loss mode you may experience some "detox" symptoms like headaches, chills, flu-like symptoms, lack of energy, dry lips, loose bowel movements…to name a few. Be sure to check in with your doctor if you experience any symptoms you are concerned about.

   - While it is typical to start losing weight in the first week (again depending on the state you started, how quickly you implement the changes and how consistent you are with them), if you don't lose weight in the first 4 weeks there is nothing to be concerned about.

5. **What is "detox"?**

- "Detox" is a very loose term I use to describe when the body is specifically focused on fat loss or is in what I call "weight loss mode". Detox happens naturally in the body; therefore, it doesn't need any help. This is why I'm not a fan of detox kits, detox juice or juice cleanses. When it comes to detox and helping the body get the fat out, there is nothing you need to do other than follow The Program. The changes in food, the design of the food plan formula, and the process of releasing fat is what causes the body to react and go into detox. We will be discussing "detox" or "weight loss mode" in more detail later.

6. **Should I be concerned if my weight isn't moving?**

- No. This is a 12-week process systematically designed to address why the body is feeling a need to store fat and make it so you can lose weight in a sustainable way… and it's a process that works if you follow The Plan.

- Please try not to stress over the little ups and downs on the scale and if you are not losing right away. If you are doing everything you need to do, then it will all come together as we move forward.

7. **What about medications and health issues, how will they affect me and do I need to do anything special to compensate or adjust?**

- We will be talking more about this as we move forward but for now focus on the basics, regardless of health issues or medications. The suggestions I have made are beneficial to everyone, as they are safe and sound and designed to get your body functioning more optimally by giving it what it needs and being consistent long enough for it to make change. If you have concerns, be sure to check in and work with your doctor along the way.

8. **Do I have to watch every Facebook Live video?**

- Although they are beneficial and informative, they are not a mandatory part of the process. You can choose to watch some, all, or none. They are posted in the Group under Guides so are always available for you to access.

9. **What if you have a question about the program or plan?**

- The Support Group should be your first source for information. It is also the place where you are to ask any questions you have day to day.

THE FOOD PLAN

The Food Plan is designed to stimulate your digestive system, increase nutrient absorption, decrease insulin levels, and give the body the resources it needs to make change. The goal is to be as consistent as possible to allow the body to react and adjust to the Food Plan. You are to eat all meals and snacks, even if you are not hungry you still need to eat a small token amount.

You will be following the Food Plan for the next few weeks and as we progress, we will be making slight changes to it week to week. So, it's key to be as consistent as possible as soon as possible.

Although it's important to eat the suggested categories of food (protein, veg, fruit etc.) at meal and snack times, the variety and sources are up to you. Be sure to review the many examples given in the Grocery List and Meal ideas Post.

THE BASIC FOOD PLAN:

FIRST THING - Warm lemon water and/or apple cider vinegar (Wait 5-10 minutes to have coffee or tea or breakfast)

BREAKFAST - Protein is the focus

SNACK #1 - Fruit on its own

LUNCH - Vegetables are the focus with added protein, leafy greens, and healthy fats. Add in grains and heavier carbs when needed.

SNACK #2 - Raw veggies, can add dips, cheese or nut butters (can be cooked if needed)

SNACK #3 - Nuts and/or seeds (see individual breakdown below for alternatives if needed)

DINNER - Protein heavy with added vegetables, leafy greens, and healthy fats.

The time between all meals and snacks should be anywhere from 30 mins to no more than 3.5 hours. It's important to keep the order of the food, but the timing between meals and snacks can change day to day.

Let's break it down and go into more detail...

LEMON/ACV WATER

Lemon Water = juice of half a lemon or 2 tbsp juice in as much warm water as you like.

ACV (apple cider vinegar containing "the mother") = 1 tablespoon in as much water as you need to get it down. If you are just starting out, you may want to start with 1 tsp and work your way up.

WHY?

Warm lemon water first thing in the morning promotes hydration and helps to stimulate your digestive system. You can use fresh lemons or bottled lemon juice as long as it is all-natural.

Another option, or in addition to the lemon water, is Apple Cider Vinegar. If you suffer from acid reflux and other digestive issues, it can be very beneficial to add in. It's also beneficial for anyone who has had their gallbladder removed.

Both are beneficial in their own ways. You can take one or the other or both. This is not "make or break" but more of an added bonus, especially if you suffer from known digestive issues.

BREAKFAST PROTEIN HEAVY

Breakfast is not the most important meal of the day; however, it can be greatly beneficial when trying to lose weight.

WHY?

When you wake up, you are already full of energy from what you ate the day before. So, you don't need to eat breakfast to gain energy.

That's why you have the option of skipping it, carrying on with your day, then going to your morning fruit snack. With that said, there is absolutely a benefit to eating it. Starting your day with a high protein breakfast is a great way to "break the fast" and get your body working harder from the get-go.

It pains me to say it...but that means burning more calories throughout your day! (And NO we still don't count calories!)

It's ideal to eat breakfast within 2.5 hours of waking. However, this is not a hard and fast rule. If you wake up at 5 am and you are not active or exercising you can still eat breakfast as late as 9 am and be fine. If you get up later, that gives you less time to have breakfast before your snack, so you might skip breakfast and go straight to snack.

We will be adding in bonus snacks to help fill in the blanks for those of you who are up early, are more active, or do shift work. For now, play around with the timing of your breakfast to figure out what's best for you.

SNACK #1: FRUIT ON ITS OWN.

Why fruit and why on its own?

Normally, it is a good idea to combine your carbs with a protein and fat which can help minimize the amount of insulin needed to convert the food you eat into energy.

Which may have you confused and wondering why we are eating the fruit on its own?!

Whether you have breakfast or not, by mid-morning, your glycogen (energy) reserves are starting to deplete. The goal is to replenish those energy stores before the body has to dip into, and utilize, your emergency fat reserves. When the body is forced to dip into its fat reserves, that sends a message to the body that you need to store fat. Which is something we are ultimately trying to avoid. So, by having fruit on its own, you are able to replenish those stores easily.

In the weeks to come, we will be making changes to your morning snack, but for now, you can have one or any combo of fruits. Fruit cups, frozen fruit, and applesauce are fine as long as they have no added sugar. Bananas are a little higher in sugar but are a great addition for anyone who is more active or in need of potassium due to leg cramps while sleeping.

LUNCH: VEG IS THE FOCUS (COOKED OR RAW) WITH PROTEIN, LEAFY GREENS (COOKED OR RAW), AND HEAVIER CARBS IF YOU FEEL THE NEED FOR THEM.

Why vegetable heavy?

Vegetables are carbohydrates, which are "energy foods". You want to eat those earlier in the day so your body has time to use them throughout the day.

If you feel you need a little more "oomph". This is also when you might want to add in some heavier carbs such as whole grains like rice or quinoa or carb-heavy veggies like squash or potatoes.. These carbs are better eaten at lunch so your body has all day to use up the energy from them.

Side note: Leafy greens do not count as vegetables on this plan so if you are having a salad, be sure to load up on vegetables!

SNACK #2: RAW VEGGIES

Raw veggies can be very hard to digest, which makes them the perfect food for the first afternoon snack and after a bigger meal.

If you find you get bloated or have a hard time digesting raw veggies, that can be a sign you are low in digestive enzymes. If you need, you can cook or steam them but do so temporarily with the goal to work your way up to eventually eating them raw.

You can eat any raw veggies you like and do not need to worry about getting in a huge variety. You can stick to the ones you do like.

You can also add natural dressings or dips like hummus or guacamole. You can also add cheese or nut butter to make your veg snack more nutrient rich.

Pickles or fermented food like kimchi or sauerkraut also work! You could also do a salad and use leafy greens as long as it's loaded up with raw veg.

Keep in mind, even if you add raw veg to lunch, you will still need the afternoon snack.

SNACK #3: NUTS AND/OR SEEDS

Nuts and seeds ideally should have no added oil or salt.

Nuts and seeds are even harder to digest than raw veggies, which is why they make the perfect afternoon snack.

Try to keep the number of nuts you eat to a maximum of approximately 25 pieces and seeds to one shot glass full. You can have one or the other, or both. They can be very hard to digest, so eating too many can lead to digestive upset. This limit isn't suggested because of calories or fat.

Nuts and seeds are even harder to digest than raw veggies, which is why they make the perfect afternoon snack. Around 3-4pm, the body is naturally wired to take a dip in energy. What the body is really looking for is a nap. Other places in the world refer to this as a siesta and take time to snooze. Because most of us can't just take a nap during the day, this is where people go looking for sugar or caffeine as a pick-me-up.

By adding in the nuts and or seeds, you are keeping your digestive system stimulated and working hard, which helps to keep your energy up. The protein and fat from the nuts and seeds also helps to give you more sustaining energy, which will have you feeling more satisfied leading up to and going into dinner.

This helps keep your digestive system working hard to process and break down your larger meal and will also help prevent you from overeating your dinner.

You can also add nuts and or seeds to your meals. If you do, keep in mind you still need to eat your Nut & Seed Snack.

If you find them hard to digest, you can roast them or soak them. If you can't eat nuts due to allergies, you can stick to seeds. If you can't have either due to allergies or preparation for a procedure, the alternatives are dairy such as cheese or yogurt, olives or beans like chickpeas, edamame, black beans etc. Please Note: these alternatives are to be used as a last resort and nuts and/or seeds are the best choice.

BOTH SNACKS MUST BE EATEN IN THAT ORDER

DINNER: PROTEIN IS THE FOCUS WITH VEGETABLES (COOKED OR RAW), LEAFY GREENS (COOKED OR RAW), AND HEALTHY FATS.

Given that it's at the end of the day, try to think of dinner as more of a top-up rather than a need for fuel. Ideally, dinner "should" be the smallest meal of the day, especially if eating after dark when our bodies are naturally winding down to get ready for sleep. Most of us were raised in a culture where dinner was the biggest meal, and this habit is hard to break, but as you work through this Program, you will start to notice your appetite for a larger dinner will decrease.

Alternatively, there might be times where you won't be very hungry for dinner, but you still need to have a token amount. In this case, some protein with a bit of leafy greens would work.

You can add heavier carbs IF you feel you need them like if you are being very active into the night.

Try to eat dinner as early as possible. Eating too late will prevent the body from following through on its wind down process, which will mess with your body's ability to get the deep REM and sleep it needs to make change.

After dinner snack: best if you can avoid it, but if you need a little something to take the edge off, you can have some air popped popcorn with butter and sea salt. Keep in mind we will be suggesting eliminating this altogether in the weeks to come.

You can also have your favourite herbal teas in the evening that can help when breaking the nighttime snacking habit.

THE GOAL:

Keep things simple and routine. Don't overthink it, it is a process, and everything will come together in time.

I'm not concerned about portion sizes or weighing or measuring food. You will find as you go along, portions will adjust on their own and you will become very in tune with what your body needs.

This first week is all about taking the time to understand the process and making the changes you need to make. Be sure to ask any questions you have along the way!

For more information, be sure to check out the Food Plan FAQs.

Please take time to head over to the Facebook Group and watch the quick video that accompanies this post.

FAQS - THE FOOD PLAN

Here are some of our most popular questions asked about the Food Plan.

1. **Do I need to follow the plan exactly and do I need to eat all the meals and snacks even if I'm not hungry?**

   - Yes! This is super key! For best results do not deviate, improvise, or skip any meals or snacks. They are all equally important and for a rhyme and a reason. The only meal you don't need to eat is breakfast as outlined in the plan.

2. **How far apart should my meals and snacks be?**

   - Anywhere from 30 minutes to 3.5 hours is fine. The order of food is important, but the timing between meals and snacks can change day to day.

BREAKFAST

1. **Should I have both lemon water and apple cider vinegar?**

   You can have one or the other or both. You can also have them together as in your ACV in your lemon water.

2. **Can I use lime instead of lemon in my morning drink?**

   Yes, you can.

3. **Can I take ACV gummies?**

   Supplements in gummy form do not provide the same benefits as taking the real thing. We don't recommend them.

4. **Can I use bottled lemon juice for my morning lemon water?**

   Yes, you can, as long as it's made with all-natural ingredients.

5. **Can I drink coffee or tea?**

   Yes, coffee and tea are totally on plan.

6. **Does coffee and tea count towards water intake?**

   Yes, all beverages except for alcohol count towards water intake.

7. **Can I have cream and sugar in my coffee?**

   Yes, you can have cream or creamers as long as they contain all-natural ingredients and are not too high in sugar. Sugar is fine. Look for raw, or organic cane. You can also use honey or maple syrup. Keep sugar to a minimum.

8. **Can I have Stevia or Monk fruit sweetener?**

Although these are better quality sweeteners, it is best to use real sugar, honey, or maple syrup.

9. **Do I have to be consistent with eating or not eating breakfast?**

No, you can eat breakfast some days and not others.

10. **Can I have protein shakes?**

I am not a fan of liquid nutrients. Especially when trying to lose weight. You want your body to work hard to digest and process its food. Especially right now while we are preparing the body for weight loss. If you insist on keeping them in, be sure to use protein powder that contains all-natural ingredients and is low in sugar. Add little to no fruit and add in some healthy fat like avocado, nut butter, coconut oil etc.

LUNCH

1. **Do I have to have salad every day?**

Definitely not. You can have a vegetable heavy meal prepared any way you like. Soup, stir fry, roasted vegetables, raw vegetables etc. with added protein and leafy greens.

2. **Can I add fruit at lunch?**

Yes, you can. Just keep it minimal.

3. **What if I'm on the road and have to stop at a fast-food restaurant?**

Most fast-food places these days have healthier options such as salads, soups, chilis, etc. These are your best bets. You can also have a sandwich or a wrap and just eat what's inside. It's okay to not be perfect every time. Sometimes life just happens so make the best choices with what you have.

4. **Can I use rice paper wrappers?**

You can, but keep in mind rice paper wrappers and rice noodles have the same effect on the body as pasta so best to avoid right now or keep to a minimum.

DINNER

1. **Can I use frozen vegetables?**

Yes, they are great for convenience. Canned ones are also fine.

2. **What about plant-based meat substitutes like Beyond Meat?**

You can, but keep it to a minimum. Many contain processed ingredients so look for quality ingredients.

3. **Can I cook with oil?**

Yes, you can use butter and oil. Choose higher quality oils such as olive oil, avocado oil, and coconut oil.

4. **Can I have potatoes or rice with dinner?**

You can, although these heavier carbs are best eaten at lunch.

5. **Can I have pasta made with Konjack, black beans, quinoa etc.**

Best to avoid any kind of pasta. Even when made with other ingredients it is still a processed product and not a whole food. No matter what the pasta is made from, it will still have your insulin levels up, which we are trying to avoid.

6. **Can I have breakfast foods for dinner?**

When it comes to eggs or things like tofu or beans then yes. But things like yogurt, cereals and oatmeal aren't the right kinds of protein for dinner at this time. There will come a time when you can have those at dinner.

7. **Can I have wine with dinner?**

Yes, alcohol is totally fine to have. You just want to drink extra water to compensate for dehydration (1 cup per drink).

8. **Can I use flour to thicken a sauce?**

Yes, small amounts of flour for thickening or breading are totally fine.

9. **Can I eat breaded meats, vegetables etc.?**

Yes, breading is totally fine.

10. **When is the best time to eat dinner?**

You want to eat dinner as early as possible and ideally before it starts getting dark.

What if I'm not hungry for dinner?

This will happen. You still want to have a token amount. In this case, some protein and leafy greens will do the trick. Further on in the process you will be able to skip dinner if you want to.

SNACKS

1. **Can I eat frozen or canned fruit for the fruit snack?**

    Yes. Fresh is better but if you choose canned or frozen, look for all natural with no added sugar.

2. **If I have fruit with breakfast, do I still need to eat fruit for the morning snack?**

    Yes. Fruit should be eaten on its own, mid-morning, regardless of whether or not you had some at breakfast.

3. **Can I have dried fruit for the fruit snack?**

    It's not ideal but if you are in a pinch, such as on the road and stuck without any other option, it's fine once in a while.

4. **Can I have more than one type of fruit, like a fruit salad?**

    Yes, any combination of fruit is fine as long as it's only fruit.

5. **Do I have to eat my veg snack if I'm still full from lunch?**

    Yes, it is key to get in all meals and snacks. If you are not hungry, you still want to eat a token amount, a few bites, to stimulate digestion.

6. **Can I have a dip with my veggies?**

    Yes, you can use dips or have with cheese, nut butter, olives or any type of healthy fat.

7. **Can I have sauerkraut or kimchi for the raw veg snack?**

    Yes, fermented foods are excellent for gut health and considered a raw veg on plan.

8. **Can I have pickles for the raw veg snack?**

    Yes, any kind of pickled vegetables work for veg snacks.

9. **What if I have problems digesting nuts and seeds?**

    If you have trouble digesting nuts and seeds you can soak and/or roast them to make them easier to digest.

10. **What if I'm allergic to nuts?**

    If you can't eat nuts due to allergies, you can stick to seeds. If you can't have either due to allergies or preparation for a procedure, the alternatives are: dairy, such as cheese or yogurt, olives, or beans like chickpeas, edamame, black beans etc. Please Note: these alternatives are to be used as a last resort as nuts and/or seeds are the best choice.

11.   **Do I eat both nuts and seeds or just one?**

You can have one or the other or both.

12.   **Can I switch out the snacks for other things or change the order?**

No. The snacks suggested are for a reason that goes far beyond just eating well. For optimal results, eat the suggested snacks at the suggested times

LET'S TALK MEAL IDEAS

Following meal plans isn't really our thing. Although we are telling you what to eat and when, within certain categories, the choices within those categories are up to you.

As we move through the 12 weeks, the goal is to get you to a place where you are very in tune with your body's cues and signals - when to eat, what to eat, and how much.

As far as portions go, right now, the goal is to eat to satisfaction. That will be different for everyone. For example, some may need 3 eggs for breakfast and others one. When it comes to portions, it's always about what you feel and not how big or small your portions look. Trust the process and follow as directed for best results. DO NOT purposefully try to reduce your portion sizes to try and speed up the process. This will backfire on you down the road.

BREAKFAST

Examples of higher protein breakfast: keep in mind these are not your only options, just some examples to get you started.

Eggs - Eggs are the best bang for your buck and by far the #1 recommendation for a high protein breakfast! Have them on their own, cooked any way you like, or with sautéed veggies, meat, cheese, a salad, small amounts of fruit, avocado etc.

Leftovers - Breakfast doesn't have to be breakfast-type food. You can also use leftovers you have in your fridge i.e. leftover meat or fish, a soup, stew, or chili. Some refried beans with avocado and salsa are some examples.

Tofu Or Tempeh - Baked, scrambled, omelets etc.

High Protein Cereal - Made with whole grains and seeds like Qia or Holy Crap brands.

Yogurt Or Cottage Cheese - Greek yogurt tends to be highest in protein. Avoid low or no fat. Add hemp hearts, nuts, nut butter and/or seeds to bump up the protein. A small amount of fruit is also okay. You can have plain or flavoured as long as it is made with natural ingredients. Added sugar is fine but watch the quantities as some brands are much higher in sugar. The higher the sugar, the higher the fat and protein content should be. Remember that we are trying to reduce insulin levels, so choosing lower to no sugar yogurts is ideal.

Chia Seed Pudding - With added hemp hearts, nuts, seeds etc. to bump up the protein.

Non-dairy Yogurt - The same as with regular yogurt, you want to add the extra toppings to bump up the protein. Coconut yogurt is low in protein so not the best option while on the program as a breakfast in itself but can be added to things like oatmeal.

Oatmeal - With added hemp hearts, nuts, nut butter and/or seeds for extra protein. You can also add high fat yogurt or other dairy/non-dairy milk or cream. Fruit and things like honey or maple syrup are fine in small amounts.

High Protein Pancakes are fine on occasion. But be mindful of what you are topping them with and be sure to add some hemp hearts or nuts/seeds.

A Note About Bread:

You can still lose weight while eating bread, but it can slow the process. If you choose to have it, look for Ezekiel bread in the freezer section at your grocery or health food store. If you can't find Ezekiel, look for other sprouted grain breads or darker denser breads that are high in protein and fiber and made with all-natural ingredients. Keep it to a minimum and have it at breakfast OR lunch. Not both.

LUNCH

Here are some examples for lunch. Keep in mind you want to have the main part of your lunch be vegetables. They can be cooked or raw and the same applies for greens.

You can also add in some heavier veggies or grains/rice if you feel the need for more oomph to your meal. Also, be sure to add in healthy fats.

Here are a few ideas to get you started.

Salad - Lunch doesn't always have to be salad, but it is a go-to for many and easy for packed lunches. Not all salads are made equal. For example, a piece of chicken on top of a Caesar salad isn't the best choice. Load up your salads with lots of veggies and things like avocado, olives, nuts, seeds, cheeses, meat, fish, beans, tofu etc. to bump up the nutrients. You can also add in grains or heavier carbs if you feel you need them.

Soup, Stew, Chili, Curry, Stir Fry - These one-pot wonders can be a life saver! You can make big batches and freeze for quick and easy meals. They can be with or without meat. Check the tips below for ideas of how to balance out the meal when necessary.

Lettuce Wraps - Use large lettuce leaves or other leafy greens to wrap up your fave sandwich fillings. Perfect for on the go!

Leftovers From Dinner - Use your leftovers for a quick and easy lunch.

Mix And Match - Lunch doesn't have to be a sit-down meal. You can toss some snack-like things into a container or onto a plate. Things like meats, cheese, boiled eggs, beans, olives, pickles, veggie sticks and dip (hummus adds protein). Add a few green leaves and you're all set!

Don't Like To Cook or Don't Have Time? - There are lots of prepared foods that fit into the plan. Check the ingredients list and look for quality. Avoid things like hydrogenated oil, MSG, artificial flavours and colours. Check the freezer section, the soup isle, the fresh made salads section etc.

DINNER

Eat dinner as early as possible to make sure your body is no longer focused on digesting food when it's winding down for sleep. There might be times you won't be very hungry for dinner, but for now, you still need to have a token amount. In this case, some protein with a bit of leafy greens would work.

There are countless possibilities for dinner but here are some ideas to get you started.

Meat, Poultry, Fish or Seafood - Grill it, bake it, bread it (yes you can use breading!), fry it (yes you can fry too!) Add your favourite veg on the side with some leafy greens (cooked or raw).

Tofu, Tempeh, Beans and Lentils - If you are looking for plant-based protein options, these are the best. Marinated tofu or tempeh, grilled, baked, or fried. Sauté some beans or lentils with veggies and seasoning or make a soup or chili.

Eggs - Eggs make a quick, light, and easy dinner. An omelet with spinach and mushrooms covers all the bases. Or eggs, any style, with some sautéed veg or a salad. Or make a Frittata and have it for breakfast, lunch, AND dinner!

Curry, Chili, Soup, Stew, Stir Fry - If you are used to having rice with your curries and stir fries, try using cauliflower rice instead.

Spaghetti Sauce - You can still make pasta for the family. Just have yours on top of zucchini noodles, cauliflower rice or cooked white beans instead!

Tacos - Put all your favourite taco fillings on a bed of leafy greens instead of in a shell or wrap.

Rotisserie Chicken - Pick up a rotisserie chicken (or 2!) from your grocery store. It's easy and convenient.

Don't Like to Cook Or Don't Have Time? - There are lots of prepared foods that fit into the plan. Check the ingredients list and look for quality. Avoid things like hydrogenated oils, artificial flavours and colours. Check the freezer section, the soup aisle, the fresh made salads section etc.

TIPS TO BALANCE THINGS OUT

HOW TO ADD EXTRA PROTEIN WITHOUT USING MEAT:

- Hemp hearts
- Nuts and/or seeds or nut butter
- Beans such as Kidney or Chickpeas
- Lentils
- Tofu
- Nutritional Yeast

- Protein powder
- Cheese or other dairy such as yogurt or cream.
- Eggs - a boiled egg with a salad makes a perfect lunch!

HOW TO ADD LEAFY GREENS:

- Have a side salad.
- Add any leafy green to your bowl or plate and add the rest (such as a soup) on top.
- Add leafy greens to the recipe such as in a soup, stew, chili or stir fry that doesn't include it. A handful of baby spinach and you are done!
- Simply pop a handful into your mouth and away you go!
- Use them as a wrap.
- Sauté a big bunch of heartier greens such as kale, collard greens, Swiss chard, Bok Choy etc. with some butter and garlic and keep in the fridge to add to any meal.

HOW TO ADD IN HEALTHY FATS:

- Use natural oils and dressings.
- Add avocados, nuts, and seeds.
- Quality cheeses.
- Fish like salmon and fresh tuna twice a week.

BREAKFAST RECIPES

EASY HOMEMADE EGG BITES

PREP & COOK TIME: 40 minutes   **SERVINGS**: 12 pieces

Homemade egg bites are a perfect make-ahead breakfast and a great way to use up leftover vegetables and other ingredients.

INGREDIENTS

EGG BASE

- 10 large eggs
- 1/4 cup plain yogurt or sour cream, full fat
- Salt and pepper to taste

SPICY RED PEPPER & PEPPER JACK

- 1 cup red pepper, small dice
- 1 cup pepper jack cheese, grated or cubed
- your favorite hot sauce, to taste

BROCCOLI & SMOKED CHEDDAR

- 1 cup broccoli, cooked, chopped into small pieces
- 1 cup smoked cheddar, grated
- 1 tbsp grainy Dijon mustard

INSTRUCTIONS

1. Preheat oven to 325°F. Generously grease a 12-cup muffin tin and place inside a larger baking pan.

2. Divide your chosen ingredients between the cups, they should be about 2/3 full.

3. Whisk together eggs, yogurt, salt, and pepper and pour evenly over each cup.

4. Pour about one to two inches of hot tap water into a larger pan. Grease a piece of foil large enough to cover the pan and cover with the greased side down. *If you don't have a larger pan, you can bake these directly in the oven leaving off the greased foil. Check for doneness after 15 minutes.*

5. Bake for 25-30 minutes or until set. Remove from the oven and remove the muffin tin from the pan. Let cool. Use a butter knife to loosen the pan. Serve warm or refrigerate or freeze for later.

STORAGE: Let cool completely and store, covered, in the fridge for 5 days. Or wrap individually and store in the freezer for up to 3 months. Let thaw in the fridge overnight.

SUBSTITUTIONS: Use any combination of vegetables or cheese you like.

HAVE IT FOR LUNCH OR DINNER: These make a perfect protein addition to any veggie packed lunch with some leafy greens! Eggs are great for dinner! Serve with a side salad or just some leafy greens

NOTES:

HIGH PROTEIN OVERNIGHT OATS

PREP TIME: 5 minutes   **SERVINGS:** 1

Overnight oats are an easy make-ahead breakfast! With all the extra add-ins this recipe packs a big protein punch! Rolled oats are the best for overnight oats. Quick cooking or instant oats will become mushy so best to avoid. Steel cut oats will have a harder texture and be less creamy.

INGREDIENTS

- ½ cup rolled oats
- ½ cup dairy or non-dairy milk
- 2 tbsp nut or seed butter
- 1 tbsp hemp hearts
- 2 tsp chia seeds

OPTIONAL TOPPINGS

- 1 tbsp chopped nuts
- 1 tbsp pumpkin or sunflower seeds
- 1 tsp maple syrup or honey
- Small amount of fruit
- Extra milk
- Unsweetened coconut

INSTRUCTIONS

1. In a glass jar or a bowl, combine oats, nut butter, hemp hearts, and chia seeds. Add a splash of the milk and mix everything together. Add in the rest of the milk and stir to combine.

2. Cover and refrigerate overnight, or up to 5 days.

3. Serve warm or cold. You can warm it up in the microwave. Heat in small increments, stirring often, until it's the temperature you like.

4. Top with chopped nuts, seeds, and fruit if using. Drizzle with maple syrup or honey if using.

STORAGE: Will keep for up to 5 days.

MAKE IT VEGAN: Use non-dairy milk such as almond, coconut or cashew.

MAKE IT NUT FREE: Use seed butter instead of nut butter and add extra seeds instead of the chopped nuts as a topping.

NOTES:

KILLER GRAIN & SEED CEREAL

Looking for a high protein breakfast to start your day off right that doesn't involve eggs, dairy or gluten? Here's the recipe you've been waiting for!

PREP & COOK TIME: 20 minutes   **SERVINGS:** 32

INGREDIENTS

TOASTED QUINOA

- 1 cup quinoa, rinsed well and drained
- 4 cups water
- 1 tbsp olive, avocado, coconut, or grapeseed oil
- 1/2 tsp salt

KILLER GRAIN & SEED CEREAL

- 1 cup toasted quinoa
- 1 cup chia seeds
- 1 cup raw buckwheat, whole kernels, or groats
- 1 cup hemp hearts/seeds

SUGGESTED TOPPINGS

- Nuts, seeds, and extra hemp hearts
- Coconut, almond, soy milk, or any milk or cream you like
- Unsweetened toasted coconut
- Yogurt
- Nut butter
- Any type of fruit

INSTRUCTIONS

FOR THE TOASTED QUINOA

1. Rinse quinoa in a mesh sieve over cold running water for about 2 minutes. Let drain.

2. Bring 4 cups of water to a boil and add quinoa. Turn down to a simmer and cook for 10 minutes. Drain well.

3. Turn the oven broiler to high and position a rack in the top third of the oven.

4. Put well drained quinoa back in the pot and mix in olive oil and salt. Spread thinly and evenly on a baking sheet.

5. Broil for 8-10 minutes (times may vary depending on your oven). Watch it carefully and stir halfway through. You will hear it pop and it will start to toast. Keep a very close eye in the last half of broiling. There should be no moisture left so if necessary lower the oven rack and toast a little longer until it is dry and crispy. For extra insurance, turn off the oven and let the quinoa cool down in the oven.

6. When done, let cool completely on the tray. It must be cooled completely before mixing with the other ingredients.

7. Store any extra toasted quinoa in an airtight container in the fridge and use it to top breakfast cereals, yogurt, salads, grilled vegetables etc.

KILLER GRAIN & SEED CEREAL

1. Mix together all 4 ingredients and keep in an airtight container in the fridge.

2. To make cereal, add 1/4 cup of boiling water to 2 tbsp cereal mix (use more or less water for a thinner or thicker texture). Let stand, covered with a plate, for 3-5 mins or until desired softness is reached. Serve topped with any combination of the suggested toppings above or create your own!

STORAGE: Store in an airtight container in the fridge for up to 1 month.

Extra toasted quinoa is delicious on top of yogurt, other cereals, salads, grilled vegetables, popcorn etc. You will soon be addicted!

NOTES:

EASY TEX MEX TOFU SCRAMBLE

Kick-start your day with this protein packed delicious, and easy tofu scramble. You can also replace the tofu with tempeh or eggs! For the eggs, replace tofu with 4 eggs, beaten, and omit the 2 tbsp of water. Tempeh is 1:1.

PREP & COOK TIME: 20 mins   **SERVINGS:** 2

INGREDIENTS

- 175 g (6 oz) extra firm tofu
- 2 tbsp olive oil
- 1/2 tsp chili powder
- 2 tbsp water
- 1/3 cup red pepper, diced
- 1 cup mushrooms, sliced
- salt and pepper to taste

OPTIONAL TOPPINGS

- avocado slices
- salsa
- fresh cilantro
- lime wedges
- sour cream
- grated cheese

INSTRUCTIONS

1. Wrap tofu in paper towel and press under something heavy like a pot or cast-iron skillet. Press for 15 minutes. Unwrap and break up with a fork until crumbly. Set aside

2. Mix chili powder and water. Set aside.

3. Heat oil in a sauté pan over medium heat.

4. Sauté mushrooms and pepper for 3-4 minutes or until soft.

5. Push vegetables to one side of the pan and add crumbled tofu.

6. Pour "sauce" over tofu and stir to combine, leaving the vegetables separate.

7. Mix everything together and sauté for 2 more minutes or until hot. Season with salt and pepper to taste.

8. Serve immediately with your choice of toppings.

STORAGE: Leftovers can be stored in the fridge for 3 days and reheated in a pan or the microwave.

SUBSTITUTIONS: This recipe can also be made with tempeh (1:1) or by using 4 eggs.

HAVE IT FOR LUNCH OR DINNER: For lunch simply add more vegetables or serve with a side salad. For dinner just add leafy greens right into the mix or on the side.

NOTES:

LUNCH RECIPES

CURRIED RED LENTIL SOUP

Curried Red Lentil Soup is flavourful, hearty, and nutritious. It's easy to make and has been a family favourite for many years. Even your kids will love it!

PREP & COOK TIME: 45-30 minutes   **SERVINGS:** 10-12

INGREDIENTS

- 1 lg white onion. approx. 2 cups diced small
- 1 lg celery stalk. approx. 1 cup diced small
- 1 jumbo carrot, approx. 1.5 cups diced small
- 1 small, sweet potato, 2 cups diced small
- 2-3 cloves garlic, 1 tbsp minced
- 8 cups baby spinach leaves, or greens of your choice
- 1 tbsp curry powder
- 1 1/2 cups red lentils, rinsed
- 3 tbsp olive oil
- 4 cups chicken stock, low sodium
- 1-400 ml can coconut milk
- 1/2 cup packed cilantro or parsley leaves. chopped
- 1/2 lemon, juice of
- Salt and pepper to taste

INSTRUCTIONS

1. Peel, rinse, chop and measure out all your ingredients first.

2. In a large pot, heat olive oil over medium high heat. Add onions and cook, stirring occasionally, for 3-5 minutes or until soft and translucent. Turn down the heat if they are browning before softening.

3. Add the celery, carrot, sweet potato, lentils, and garlic, stir to combine. Add curry powder and continue stirring for one minute.

4. Stir in stock and coconut milk. Increase the heat and bring to a boil. Once boiling, reduce heat and simmer. covered, for 15 minutes.

5. Stir in spinach. It will seem like a lot, but it wilts and reduces as it cooks. Cover and simmer for 5 more minutes.

6. Remove from heat and add lemon juice and cilantro or parsley. Add salt and pepper to taste. You can also add a bit more stock or water if it's too thick for your liking.

STORAGE: This soup will keep in the fridge for 5 days or in the freezer for up to 6 months.

SUBSTITUTIONS: You can use any type of lentils but cooking time may need to increase slightly. Continue cooking until the lentils are soft. Use vegetable stock instead of chicken stock and heavy cream instead of coconut milk.

HAVE IT FOR DINNER: This soup is well balanced with both vegetables and protein but if you'd like to bump up the protein a bit more, sprinkle with hemp hearts, toasted seeds or nuts. Top it with a dollop of sour cream or plain Greek yogurt or a boiled egg!

MAKE IT VEGETARIAN: Replace the chicken stock with vegetable stock.

NOTES:

QUINOA STUFFED PEPPERS

These Quinoa Stuffed Peppers are my take on a Greek Salad baked in a pepper. They make a well-balanced lunch and are delicious warm or cold!

PREP AND COOK TIME: 45-60 mins   **SERVINGS:** 8 half peppers

INGREDIENTS

FOR THE PEPPERS

- 1/2 cup quinoa, uncooked
- Olive oil for coating peppers and frying vegetables
- 4 large bell peppers, any colours
- 1 cup chopped red onion
- 2 large cloves garlic, minced
- 1 medium zucchini, cut into small cubes
- 1 cup chopped tomato
- 1/2 cup Kalamata olives, pitted and chopped
- 1/4 cup each fresh basil and parsley, chopped
- 10 balls mini bocconcini cheese, cut in half
- Salt and pepper to taste
- 100 g feta cheese
- 1/2 lemon

SIMPLE TZATZIKI SAUCE

- 1, 3-inch piece cucumber
- 1 cup plain Greek yogurt
- 1 tbsp chopped. fresh dill
- 1/4 lemon, juiced
- 1 sm. clove garlic, minced
- Salt and pepper to taste

INSTRUCTIONS

FOR THE PEPPERS

1. Rinse quinoa in a sieve under cold water for at least 2 minutes. Bring a pot of water to a boil. Add salt and cook quinoa for 12-15 minutes. Strain and rinse under cold water. Leave it in the strainer and set aside.

2. Turn BBQ on to high heat. Or if using the oven, preheat to 450 degrees F.

3. Cut peppers in half lengthwise and remove the seeds and core. Leave the tops on. In a large bowl, toss with olive oil, salt, and pepper.

4. Place peppers on the grill cut side down. Cook for 8-10 minutes on that side or until the edges are charred. Turn and cook for an additional 4-5 minutes. They are done when just starting to soften, but not limp. Cooking time will vary depending on your BBQ. Remove from the grill to a tray and let cool. Alternatively roast, cut side down, on a lined baking tray, in a preheated oven for 8-10 minutes or until just beginning to soften.

5. In a large sauté pan, heat 1 tbsp olive oil over medium-high heat. Add red onion and cook for 2-3 minutes. Add garlic and zucchini. Cook, stirring for 2-3 minutes more. Remove from heat and add cooked quinoa, tomatoes, olives, fresh herbs, and bocconcini cheese. Mix well. Season with salt and pepper to taste.

6. Preheat or reduce the oven to 350°F.

7. In an oiled baking dish, place the peppers together snugly but with enough room to add filling. Fill each pepper generously. At this point peppers can be covered and refrigerated overnight if made ahead.

8. In a preheated oven, bake for 15 minutes or until filling is warmed through. Remove from the oven, squeeze with lemon juice and sprinkle with crumbled feta cheese. These can be served warm or at room temperature.

SIMPLE TZATZIKI SAUCE

1. Grate the cucumber and place in a sieve over a bowl. Sprinkle it with salt. Let stand for a minimum of 15 minutes and up to an hour. Squeeze out any excess water.

2. In a medium bowl combine the drained cucumber with yogurt, dill, garlic, lemon juice, salt, and pepper to taste. Stir together. This sauce will keep in the fridge for one week.

STORAGE: Filling can be made ahead and stored, covered, in the fridge for up to 24 hours. Peppers can be made in advance. After you finish stuffing, cover, and refrigerate for up to 24 hours. Proceed to baking instructions. Finished peppers will keep in the fridge, covered, for 5 days. Tzatziki sauce will keep for one week in the fridge.

HAVE IT FOR DINNER: These peppers make a great side dish to your favourite protein. Don't forget the leafy greens!

ADD LEAFY GREENS: Serve these peppers on a bed of greens or with a side salad.

NOTES:

ROASTED VEGETABLE SALAD WITH SPICED CHICKPEAS & TAHINI DRESSING

This makes a large batch for you to enjoy for a few days. Mix and match the components by serving the vegetables as a side with dinner, tossing chickpeas on any dish where you want to bump up the protein, and using the dressing as a dip or drizzled on nearly anything! Tahini and chickpeas add enough protein to make this a balanced lunch.

PREP & COOK TIME: 1-hour   **SERVINGS:** 6-8

INGREDIENTS

- 2 medium carrots, peeled and cut into 2" sticks, 2 cups
- 1 medium sweet potato, peeled and diced, 2 cups
- 1 red bell pepper, cored and sliced ½ inch thick, 1 cup
- 1 small head cauliflower, cut into small florets, 3 cups
- 10 radishes, rinsed and cut in half or quarters depending on size, 1 cup
- 8 Brussels sprouts, halved or quartered depending on size, 2 cups
- 4 tbsp olive oil
- 1 tsp salt
- freshly ground black pepper to taste

SPICED CHICKPEAS

- 2 cans (425g/15oz) chickpeas, drained, rinsed, and dried well, 4 cups
- 2 tbsp olive oil
- ½ tsp salt
- 1 tsp ground cumin
- 2 tsp chili powder
- ¼ tsp cayenne pepper

LEMON TAHINI DRESSING

- ½ cup tahini paste
- Juice of one lemon, 2-3 tbsp.
- ½ tsp salt, plus more to taste
- ¼ cup ice water

INSTRUCTIONS

SPICED CHICKPEAS

1. Preheat the oven to 400 degrees F. Line a baking tray with parchment paper.

2. Carefully dry the chickpeas, removing any loose skins. I do this by laying them on a dish towel lined tray with another towel on top and rub to dry. Place in a medium bowl and toss with olive oil and salt.

3. In a small bowl mix cumin, chili powder, and cayenne. Set aside.

4. Spread chickpeas onto a lined baking tray and roast in the oven for 15 minutes. Turn the tray and shake the chickpeas around for even cooking. Continue roasting for another 15 minutes, or until desired crispiness is reached. Meanwhile prepare the vegetables and tahini dressing.

5. Remove from the oven and toss immediately with the spices. Stir to coat and place back on the baking tray to cool. They will continue to crisp as they cool.

ROASTED VEGETABLES

1. Preheat the oven to 400 degrees F. Line 2 baking sheets with parchment paper.

2. Place all prepared vegetables into a large bowl and toss with 4 tbsp. of olive oil. Divide in half onto each tray. Don't overcrowd the vegetables or they will steam instead of roast. Sprinkle each tray with ½ tsp salt and freshly ground pepper to taste. Place in the oven and roast for 30 minutes, stirring and rotating pans halfway through cooking.

LEMON TAHINI DRESSING

1. Stir the tahini to mix in any separated oil. This will take a couple of minutes. In a medium bowl, whisk together tahini paste, lemon juice, salt, and ice water. It will appear to seize at first but as you continue whisking it will smooth out and become light in colour. If it doesn't, it needs more water. Add a teaspoon at a time until it reaches the right consistency which should barely drip from your whisk. Taste and add more salt if necessary.

ASSEMBLY

This salad can be served warm or cold. Top vegetables with spiced chickpeas and drizzled with tahini dressing. Add approximately ¼ cup of chickpeas and 2 tbsp of dressing to every 2 cups of vegetables for a balanced lunch.

STORAGE Store **roasted vegetables** in an airtight container in the refrigerator for up to 5 days. **Roasted chickpeas** are best stored loosely covered at room temperature to retain their crispiness. They will lose their crispness but will last for 4 days at room temperature. The more dried out they are the longer they will last. Store **tahini dressing** in a jar or sealed container for 2 weeks. Loosen with a bit of water, if necessary, before serving.

SUBSTITUTIONS - Use any combination of vegetables you like. Some other great additions are broccoli, mushrooms, zucchini, red onion, etc.

HAVE IT FOR DINNER: Serve this salad as a side dish to your favourite protein for dinner. Or increase the amount of chickpeas and add things like cheese, hemp heart, nuts and/or seeds.

ADD LEAFY GREENS: There are Brussels sprouts in the mix which work as both a veg and leafy green but if you are looking to bump up your leafy greens, serve on a bed of your favourite leaves or toss them up with the vegetables before serving.

NOTES:

THAI STYLE SLAW WITH PEANUT DRESSING

A crunchy and delicious Thai style slaw. It's easy to prepare and keeps for days in the fridge! This salad has everything you need for a perfectly balanced lunch on plan. Or have it for dinner as a side to your favourite protein!

PREP TIME: 30 minutes   **SERVINGS:** 6

INGREDIENTS

- 1 cup edamame beans, steamed
- 4 cups (1/2 a head) savoy cabbage, thinly sliced
- 1 bell pepper, thinly sliced
- 1 cup snow peas, thinly sliced
- 1 medium-large carrot, shredded
- 2 green onions, thinly sliced
- 1/2 cup cilantro, chopped
- 1/2 cup chopped peanuts, for garnish
- lime wedges, for garnish

PEANUT DRESSING

- 2 cloves garlic, minced
- 4 tbsp fresh squeezed lime juice
- 3 tbsp soy sauce
- 1/2 cup peanut butter, all natural
- 2 tsp avocado or olive oil
- 2 tsp brown sugar
- 1/4 tsp crushed pepper flakes
- 4 tbsp water, or more

INSTRUCTIONS

FOR THE DRESSING

1.   In a bowl, food processor, or blender, mix all ingredients. Add more water if necessary to thin. The amount of water will depend on the consistency of your peanut butter. Set aside.

FOR THE SALAD

1. Steam or blanch edamame beans for 5 minutes or until tender. Drain and run under cold water to cool after cooking.

2. Chop peanuts and set aside for garnish.

3. Slice all the vegetables using a sharp knife or mandolin. Chop cilantro. Toss everything together in a large bowl.

4. Add dressing and toss to combine.

Serve garnished with chopped peanuts and lime wedges.

STORAGE: Store, covered, in the refrigerator for up to one week. The salad will wilt as it sits but remains crunchy and delicious!

SUBSTITUTIONS: Substitute green cabbage with savoy or red cabbage, or a combination. Substitute peanut butter for almond or cashew butter. For a completely nut-free alternative try using Sunbutter which is made from sunflower seeds.

HAVE IT FOR DINNER: Serve as a side to your favourite protein!

NOTES:

DINNER RECIPES

TEMPEH AND ROASTED CHICKPEA CURRY

If you follow a plant-based diet or are looking to consume less meat, tempeh is a fantastic source of protein. Similar to tofu but with a firmer, meatier texture that has a nutty taste. It's made of fermented soybeans so it is also great for gut health!

PREP AND COOK TIME: 40 mins   **SERVINGS**: 4

INGREDIENTS

- 1 (390 ml/14 oz) can chickpeas, drained and rinsed
- 1/2 tsp ground cumin
- 1/2 tsp smoked paprika
- 1/2 tsp salt
- 1 tbsp coconut or olive oil
- 1 (250g) package tempeh, original flavour
- 1 tbsp cornstarch
- 1/2 tsp salt
- 1/2 large red onion, sliced thinly
- 1 medium to large fresh tomato, chopped
- 3 cloves fresh garlic, chopped
- 3 + 1 tbsp coconut oil
- 2 tbsp curry paste (I used Patak's hot curry paste)
- 1 (398 ml/14 oz can) full fat coconut milk
- 1 tsp sugar
- 2 cups baby spinach leaves, packed

OPTIONAL GARNISHES

- plain yogurt
- sliced red onion
- chopped fresh cilantro
- fresh lemon wedges

INSTRUCTIONS

1. Preheat the oven to 400 degrees F.

2. Toss chickpeas with cumin, smoked paprika, and salt. Place on a parchment lined baking tray and bake for 10 minutes.

3. Cut tempeh into approximately 1 cm (1/2-inch) cubes. Toss with cornstarch and 1/2 tsp. salt.

4. Prepare the onion, garlic, and tomato.

5. Heat 2 3 tbsp. coconut oil in a large sauté pan over medium-high heat. Add tempeh and fry to brown all sides. Lower heat if browning too quickly. Remove from pan to a bowl or plate.

6. Lower heat to medium-low. Add another tablespoon of coconut oil to the pan.

7. Add sliced onions and sauté until softened. 8-10 minutes.

8. Add garlic and tomatoes and stir for one minute.

9. Add tempeh, chickpeas, and curry paste. Stir to coat everything in the curry paste.

10. Add coconut milk and 1 tsp sugar. Mix everything together.

11. Increase heat and bring to a boil. Reduce heat to a simmer and continue simmering for 10 minutes or until it reaches your desired thickness.

12. Add spinach and stir until wilted.

13. Serve with your favourite rice, spaghetti squash, cauliflower rice or zucchini "noodles".

STORAGE: Store covered in refrigerator for 5 days. Freeze for 3 months.

SUBSTITUTIONS: Instead of tempeh you could use extra firm tofu, chicken, fish or shrimp. In place of spinach use any leafy green you like. Substitute curry paste with 2 tsp. curry powder.

HAVE IT FOR LUNCH: Serve with extra vegetables or a side salad for lunch. You can also add in your favourite brown or dark rice here.

SERVE WITH: Spaghetti squash, spiralized zucchini, cauliflower rice.

NOTES:

TEX-MEX CHICKEN BAKE

A quick and easy one pot meal that will soon become a family favourite! Colourful vegetables and fresh flavours will make your mouth water!

PREP & COOK TIME: 1-hour   **SERVINGS:** 4 to 6

INGREDIENTS

- 6 chicken thighs, bone-in, skin on
- 1 large white onion, peeled and diced
- 1 large red bell pepper, or any colour, diced
- 1 large zucchini, diced
- 2 large cloves garlic, finely chopped, 1 tbsp.
- 1/2 tsp ground cumin
- 1 tsp chili powder
- 1 cup fresh or frozen corn kernels
- 2 cups of your favourite salsa
- salt and pepper to taste
- fresh cilantro, one small bunch, washed and roughly chopped. Divide in two portions. One half is for garnish.
- 150 g or about 2 cups old cheddar cheese, grated
- 2-3 green onions, sliced, for garnish

OPTIONAL TOPPINGS

- Sour cream
- guacamole or avocado
- pickled jalapenos

INSTRUCTIONS

1. Preheat the oven to 400 degrees F.
2. Season chicken thighs on both sides with salt and pepper.
3. Heat olive oil in a large sauté pan over medium-high heat.

4. Add chicken thighs, skin side down and set sear, without moving them, for 4-5 minutes or until golden brown. Flip over and sear the other side for 3-4 minutes more or until golden brown.

5. Remove chicken to a large plate or dish and set aside.

6. Add diced onion to the pan with the oil and fat from the chicken. Sauté, stirring occasionally, for about 5 minutes or until soft and glossy.

7. Add diced zucchini, red pepper, garlic, cumin, and chili powder. Continue cooking and stirring occasionally for 3-4 minutes.

8. Add corn and cook for 2 more minutes. Add salsa and half the chopped cilantro. Taste and add salt and pepper as needed.

9. Bring to a boil and reduce heat to a simmer. Nestle chicken pieces into the vegetable mixture.

10. Top with grated cheddar leaving the chicken skin exposed.

11. Bake in a preheated oven for 30 minutes or until a thermometer reads 165 degrees F.

12. Top with remaining cilantro and sliced green onions.

13. Serve on its own or with rice or quinoa. Top with sour cream and/or guacamole.

STORAGE Keep covered in the fridge for 3 days or freeze for up to 3 months.

SUBSTITUTIONS - Black beans, tofu, or shrimp work well in place of chicken. Use any combination of vegetables you like. You can use boneless thighs or breasts. Cooking times may vary.

HAVE IT FOR LUNCH - Have a larger portion of vegetables than chicken/protein and serve on a bed of leafy greens.

ADD LEAFY GREENS Serve with a side salad or add 3-4 cups chopped spinach, kale, collard greens, or Swiss chard in step #7.

MAKE IT VEGETARIAN Omit the chicken and add 1 2 cans of black beans. Add the beans in step # 9. Or slice a block of firm tofu and follow the recipe as is, browning the tofu first.

NOTES:

TERIYAKI SALMON BAKE

Who doesn't love a one pan meal? This Teriyaki Salmon Bake is so easy, super nutritious, and lip-smacking good! The teriyaki sauce is delicious on any type of fish, seafood, meat, poultry, and tofu so make a big batch and keep it in the fridge for quick access.

PREP & COOK TIME: 45 minutes   **SERVINGS:** 3 or more (you can add as many filets as you like)

INGREDIENTS

- 3 salmon filets or as many as you need
- 1/2 head Napa or savoy cabbage, Bok choy or other Asian greens, chopped or sliced in large pieces
- 1 red pepper. sliced
- 1 medium carrot, thinly sliced
- 1 handful green beans or asparagus, cut into 2-inch pieces
- 2 tbsp olive or avocado oil
- 1/2 tsp salt, or to taste

TERIYAKI SAUCE

- 1/2 cup soy sauce
- 3 tbsp brown sugar
- 1 tbsp garlic, minced
- 3 tbsp mirin
- 1 tsp sesame oil
- 1/4 cup water
- 2 1/2 tsp cornstarch

OPTIONAL TOPPINGS

- toasted sesame seeds
- sliced green onions

INSTRUCTIONS

1. Preheat the oven to 400 degrees F. Place the rack in the center of the oven.

2. In a small saucepan mix together all the ingredients for the Teriyaki sauce. Bring to a boil and stir until slightly thickened. Set aside to cool.

3. Prepare all the vegetables and place in a 9" x 13" baking dish or something similar that will fit vegetables in an even layer. Drizzle with olive oil. sprinkle with salt and toss to coat.

4. Bake vegetables for 15 minutes.

5. Meanwhile, rinse salmon filets and pat dry. After 15 minutes remove vegetables from the oven and lay salmon filets on top.

6. Using about half of the Teriyaki sauce, coat the salmon and drizzle over vegetables.

7. Bake for 10 minutes. Remove from the oven and turn broil to low.

8. Brush or drizzle the remaining sauce over salmon.

9. Broil on the middle rack for 5 minutes. Check salmon for doneness. Internal temperature should read 145 degrees F. It should separate easily and be semi-translucent in the center.

10. Serve immediately. Top with toasted sesame seeds and/or sliced green onions if desired.

STORAGE: Salmon bake will keep in the fridge for 3 days. Teriyaki sauce will keep in the fridge for up to one month.

SUBSTITUTIONS: Substitute any vegetable you like including broccoli, cauliflower, Brussels sprouts, snow peas etc. Substitute Mirin with white wine or rice vinegar mixed with 3 tsp sugar.

HAVE IT FOR LUNCH: Make veggies the star of the show when having it for lunch.

ADD LEAFY GREENS: If you are looking to bump up your leafy greens you can serve on a bed of your favourite leaves.

MAKE IT VEGETARIAN: Substitute the salmon with slices of tofu marinated for 30 mins in the teriyaki sauce.

NOTES:

WHITE BEAN, SAUSAGE AND ARUGULA SOUP

White Bean Sausage and Arugula Soup is an easy and fast one pot meal that is sure to please the whole family!

PREP & COOK TIME: 1 HOUR   **SERVINGS:** 10-12

INGREDIENTS

- 1 lg white or Spanish onion, diced, about 2 cups
- 2 lg celery stalks, diced, about 1 cup
- 2-3 medium carrots, peeled and diced, about 1 cup
- 8 cloves garlic, peeled and minced
- 1 kg or 2 lbs. Italian sausage, or your favorite kind
- 6-8 cups chicken stock, homemade or store bought
- Parmesan rind, optional, and/or freshly grated Parmesan cheese
- 2 (540 ml or 18 oz) cans white beans, navy, cannellini, or kidney
- 2 cups arugula, packed. Add more to taste
- 1/2 cup chopped fresh basil
- 1-2 tbsp lemon juice
- 1-2 tsp salt
- fresh ground black pepper to taste

INSTRUCTIONS

1. Peel and dice onions, celery, carrots, and garlic.

2. Heat a large soup pot or Dutch oven over medium heat. Add 2 tbsp olive oil. Add onions, celery, carrots, and 1 tsp salt. Cook, stirring occasionally, for 8-10 minutes, or until onions are soft and translucent.

3. Meanwhile, remove casings from sausages. When vegetables are soft, add sausage and garlic. Using a wooden spoon, break up the sausage into small pieces and cook for 8-10 minutes or until the sausage is cooked and starting to brown.

4. Add chicken stock and Parmesan rind if using. Increase heat and bring to a boil. Reduce heat and simmer gently for 15 minutes.

5. Meanwhile, rinse and drain beans. Place 1/3 to 1/2 of the beans on a plate or cutting board and mash with a fork. After soup has simmered for 15 minutes add the whole and mashed beans and continue simmering for another 15 minutes.

6.   Add arugula and chopped basil. Simmer for 5 more minutes. Add more stock if you want to thin it out more. Remove from heat and add fresh lemon juice. Taste and adjust seasonings, adding more salt and/or pepper as needed.

7.   Garnish each serving with some freshly grated Parmesan cheese.

STORAGE: Store in the refrigerator for 4 days and in the freezer for 6 months.

SUBSTITUTIONS: Use any of your favourite sausages or ground meat of any kind. Substitute arugula for any leafy green such as kale, spinach, collard greens or Swiss chard.

HAVE IT FOR LUNCH: Serve a bowl with a salad or side of veggie sticks.

MAKE IT VEGETARIAN: Omit sausage and add an extra can of beans or replace sausage with crumbled up tofu or tempeh. Replace chicken stock with vegetable stock.

NOTES:

GROCERY CHECKLIST

FRUIT

Any kind of fruit or combination of fruits you like. Literally ANY kind. Fresh fruit is best but frozen and canned are fine as well. Canned fruit should be without added sugar. Avoid dried fruits for this part of the program.

- Apples
- Apricots
- Bananas
- Berries (all)
- Cherries
- Cranberries (fresh)
- Dates (fresh & Medjool)
- Fresh figs
- Grapefruit

- Grapes
- Kiwi
- Lemons
- Limes
- Mango
- Melons (all)
- Nectarines
- Oranges (all types)
- Papaya

- Peaches
- Pears
- Pineapple
- Plums
- Pomelo
- Pomegranate
- _____
- _____
- _____

VEGETABLES

Any and all vegetables are on plan. Choose vegetables for both eating raw and cooked. Add your own to the list if some are missing

- Artichokes
- Asparagus
- Bell Peppers
- Beets
- Bok Choy (veg & leafy green)
- Broccoli
- Broccoli Rabe/ Rapini (veg & leafy green)
- Brussels sprouts (veg & leafy green)
- Cabbage (veg & leafy green)
- Carrots
- Cauliflower
- Celery

- Celeriac/Celery Root
- Corn
- Cucumber
- Edamame Beans
- Eggplant
- Fennel
- Fiddleheads (veg & leafy green)
- Green beans
- Green Peas (all types)
- Hearts of palm
- Hot Peppers (all)
- Jicama
- Kimchi (veg & leafy green)
- Kohlrabi

- Leeks/Scallions
- Mushrooms (all)
- Onions (all)
- Pickled Vegetables(all)
- Radishes
- Rhubarb
- Sauerkraut (veg & leafy green)
- Spaghetti squash
- Sprouts
- Tomatoes
- Turnip & Rutabaga
- Zucchini/summer squash
- Water Chestnuts

HEAVIER VEGETABLES (IDEALLY ADDED AT LUNCH WHEN NEEDED)

- Cassava
- Parsnips
- Plantain
- Potatoes
- Pumpkin
- Squash
- Sweet potatoes/Yams
- Yucca
- _____
- _____
- _____
- _____

PROTEIN

Protein is needed at breakfast, lunch and dinner so consider each meal when making your shopping list. Always look for quality products, "raised without hormones or antibiotics" "grass-fed" "all natural" "organic" etc. Quality is key!

Plant based proteins labeled as higher protein veg should not be used as a stand-alone protein source but are great when used in combination with other protein sources.

ANIMAL

- Eggs
- Chicken (all cuts, with or without skin)
- Turkey (all cuts, with or without skin)
- Beef (all cuts)
- Pork (all cuts)
- Game Meats
- Fish (all types)
- Seafood (all types)
- Canned meat/fish

PLANT BASED

- Tofu
- Tempeh
- Edamame Beans (higher protein veg)
- Sprouts (higher protein veg)
- Lentils
- Beans/Chickpeas
- Nutritional Yeast
- Hemp Hearts/Seeds
- Nuts (all)
- NutButters(all)

KEEP TO A MINIMUM

- Bacon
- Sausages (unless all natural/good quality)
- Deli Meats look for all natural

LEAFY GREENS

Leafy greens are added as roughage. Any leafy green works and can be eaten raw or cooked.

- Arugula
- Bok Choy (veg and leafy)
- Broccoli Rabe/Rapini (veg and leafy)
- Brussels Sprouts (veg and leafy)
- Cabbage (veg and leafy)
- Chinese Broccoli (veg and leafy)
- Collard Greens
- Endive
- Fiddleheads (veg and leafy)
- Iceberg lettuce
- Kale
- Leaf Lettuce
- Mustard Greens
- Radicchio
- Romaine lettuce
- Salad Mixes (all)
- Seaweed
- Spring Mix
- Spinach
- Swiss Chard
- Watercress

GRAINS

Whole Grains are best added to lunch if you feel the need to have a little more substance. You can have them at dinner too but keep the portion size small and try not to have it every day. Also, oats and high protein cereals are fine to have at breakfast with added hemp hearts, nuts and seeds or quality protein powder, to boost protein.

- Amaranth
- Barley
- Buckwheat
- Bulgur (cracked wheat)
- Farro
- Millet
- Oats Add extra protein when having
- for breakfast (See Meal Ideas Post for more details)
- Rice - black, red, wild, brown, white or brown basmati
- Quinoa
- Sorghum
- Teff

DAIRY

<u>**Avoid low or no-fat dairy products**</u> except for milk and cream, which can be any fat content. **Always avoid artificial flavors, colors, or artificial sweeteners.**

- Add hemp hearts, nuts and seeds, nut butter or quality protein powder to yogurt to bump up the protein.

- If eating non-dairy yogurt, nut and soy based are best. Coconut yogurt contains very little protein.

- Some sugar is okay in both yogurts and coffee creamers. Just keep to a minimum and with yogurt, add extra fat/protein.

- There are far too many cheeses to list them all here.

- All cheese is fine as long as it isn't processed or containing artificial colours or flavours.

- Although there is protein in dairy products, they are not a good stand-alone protein on program so should be used with an addition of extra protein such as nuts, seeds, hemp hearts etc.

- Greek yogurt -Ideally plain and unsweetened with 2% or higher MF. If sweetened, choose higher fat.
- Non-dairy yogurts
- Cottage Cheese
- Sour cream
- Milk (any fat %)
- Cream (any fat %)
- Non-dairy milk (all)
- Kefir
- Butter
- Havarti
- Swiss
- Gouda
- Provolone
- Mozzarella
- Parmesan
- Manchego
- Blue cheese
- Brie/camembert
- White cheddar
- Goat's cheese
- Cream cheese (no artificial flavours)
- Feta
- Bocconcini

FATS

Healthy fats are an important part of weight loss. Here are some examples of healthy fats to have on hand. Adding extra healthy fats to meals bumps up the nutrient value.

- Extra Virgin Olive Oil
- Avocado Oil
- Coconut Oil
- Cold pressed canola oil
- Ghee/Clarified Butter
- Butter
- Sesame Oil
- Nut Oils
- Flax Oil
- Hemp Oil
- Avocados
- Nuts (all types)
- Coconut
- Nut Butters (all natural)
- Seeds (all types)
- Olives

MISCELLANEOUS - OPTIONAL ITEMS

When looking for condiments, sauces, dressings, or pre-packaged food items, **avoid ingredients like artificial flavor, artificial colour, hydrogenated oils.** The organic and health food sections of your grocery store or your health food store are great places to look for quality prepackaged foods.

- Bottled lemon or lime juice (100% natural)
- High quality protein powder containing all-natural ingredients if using for oats or yogurt.
- Protein grain cereals such as Qia or Holy Crap
- Salad dressings
- Bottled sauces (BBQ, curry, stir fry etc.)
- Mayonnaise

- Ketchup/mustard & other condiments
- Dips for vegetables
- Premade soups, chilis, etc.
- Any herbs and spices
- Sugar raw, organic cane, coconut, honey, maple syrup
- High fiber crackers such as Ryvita brand or equivalent
- Ezekiel bread (see Note)

A NOTE ABOUT BREAD

You can still lose weight while eating bread, but it can slow the process. If you choose to have it, look for Ezekiel bread in the freezer section at your grocery or health food store. If you can't find Ezekiel, look for other sprouted grain breads or darker denser breads that are high in protein and fiber and made with all-natural ingredients. Keep it to a minimum and have it at breakfast OR lunch. Not both.

LET'S TALK WATER

As you know, water and how much you need to drink is a hot topic when it comes to the Program. Increasing your water intake, in my experience, is one of the top things you can do to help maximize your efforts to drop fat.

Unlike traditional diets that force your body to burn fat by way of eating less or exercising more, my program uses the body's natural detox process to help the body release fat and water is key in helping that happen. The body releases fat when you pee, poo, breathe and sweat.

Lack of studies and a lot of misinformation about water and hydration has left people confused about how much they need to drink. The average person needs at least 2.7 to 3.5 liters of water for basic body functions like digestion, pumping blood through your veins, sweating, bowel movements etc. (Source: refer to original post in the group for source).

To help the body get into detox mode, you will need to drink above and beyond what it needs for basic body functions.

"Detox mode" is a loose term I use when referring to the body being specifically focused on getting the fat out. Although the body is capable of detoxing on its own, it will do so at a very slow and frustrating pace. This is why we have designed a program that will utilize and support that process.

Besides aiding in fat loss, being properly hydrated has many other health benefits such as:

- Increased energy and brain function
- Can help relieve constipation
- Increased cardiovascular health
- Increased function of muscles and joints
- Promotes healthy "glowing" skin
- Helps flush toxins from your organs
- Helps curb cravings, especially for sugar

SO HOW MUCH SHOULD I BE DRINKING?

This is a simple question with no easy answer.

Everyone requires different amounts, so you will have to play around with it to see what works for you, what helps to get you into detox and what helps keep you there. Your water intake can also change from day to day depending on many factors. Here's a list of things that can affect how much water you need above the 2.7 to 3.5 litres.

YOU NEED EXTRA WATER WHEN:

- Your body is in detox
- You are fighting an illness
- You have your period
- You take medication that causes weight gain or dehydration
- You work or live in a dry environment
- You exercise or are active enough to sweat
- You drink alcohol
- You eat salty food
- You are taller than average (over 5'5" for women, 5'9" for men)
- You have weight to lose

Since you are all trying to get rid of fat, I suggest aiming for 3.5 litres to start. You can adjust from there depending on your height, weight and other factors listed above. Some of you might find this is enough and others might find they need more.

HOW DO I KNOW I'M DRINKING ENOUGH?

- You no longer feel thirsty
- You no longer have dry mouth or lips
- Your trips to the bathroom have decreased (they will increase until you are properly hydrated)

HOW MUCH IS TOO MUCH?

Overhydration and water intoxication happen when you drink more water than your kidneys can get rid of through urine. You have a greater risk of developing water intoxication if you drink a lot of water in a short period of time. When you drink too much too fast, your kidneys can't get rid of the excess water. Your kidneys can eliminate about 5 to 7 gallons (20-28 litres) of water a day, but they can't get rid of more than 27 - 33 ounces (0.8 - 1.0 litres) per hour.

Therefore, to avoid hyponatremia (low salt in blood) or overhydration from excess water, you should not drink more than 27 - 33 ounces (0.8 - 1.0 litres) of water per hour, on average and be mindful to include salt in your diet.

WHEN INCREASING WATER INTAKE:

- Increase slowly.

- Start early and spread your water drinking throughout the day. Don't chug a large amount at once.

- To prevent low sodium levels, add a pinch of pink Himalayan, Celtic or Sea salt to your warm water and lemon or ACV in the morning. This will add in minerals and electrolytes as well as support hormone and adrenal function. Or you can purchase trace minerals to add to your water.

- When it comes to water, it's not about drinking more and more. It's about drinking enough. Do what's right for you and always consult with your doctor if you have any concerns.

TIPS TO GETTING IT IN:

- Make it fun! Make it a challenge!

- Start drinking early in your day. Most people find it easier to get the majority in the first half of the day.

- Sip, don't guzzle.

- Get a good water bottle or cup that you like to drink from.

- Track your water (and other fluids such as coffee, tea, bone broth) intake by using our Livy Method tracking app.

- Set reminders to drink.

- Add fresh or frozen fruit, cucumber slices, and/or fresh herbs or ginger.

- Stop drinking after dinner, so it doesn't mess with your sleep.

This can be the hardest part of the program but also the most important, so keep at it and do your best.

...it does get easier and if you make it a challenge it can be fun!

Once you have lost the weight, you can adjust and scale back on the amount you are drinking to maintain hydration without having to push more for the sake of weight loss.

On a final note: Tea, Coffee, soups, and essentially any other liquid (except alcohol) counts towards your water intake. Sparkling water is okay on occasion, but the majority of your water intake should be regular water.

Please take time to head over to the Facebook Group and watch the quick video that accompanies this post.

FAQS - WATER

Here are some of our most popular questions asked about water.

1.   Why so much water?

The average person needs 2.7 - 3.5 litres of water just for basic body functions like processing the food going in and going out. Because this program piggy-backs the body's natural detox response, you will need to drink above and beyond the minimum to get your body into detox mode (releasing fat).

2.   Can I drink too much?

You would really have to drink above and beyond the minimum recommended to an extreme, for there to be any detrimental side effects. However, although the kidneys can take in up to 20-28 litres of fluid per day, they cannot excrete more than 1 litre per hour. So, try not to drink more than 1 litre per hour and sip instead of guzzling.

You also want to be mindful of low sodium. When increasing water intake, be mindful to add salt to meals or add in trace minerals.

Make sure you're drinking enough for your body's needs and not just drinking as much as possible.

3.   Does it matter when I drink the water?

Try to start early in the morning and spread it out throughout the day. Drinking into the later hours can cause disruption in your sleep so better if you can be done earlier rather than later.

4.   Will I always have to drink this much water?

The extra water is only necessary while you are trying to lose weight. When maintaining your weight, you can scale back to basic requirements. The amount of water you need will fluctuate from day to day both during and after weight loss.

5.   Can I add anything to my water?

You can add fresh or frozen fruit, fresh herbs etc. Anything that is all natural, with no sugar or sweeteners added. Naturally flavoured tea also counts towards water intake.

6.   How should I keep track of my water intake?

There are many methods, so experiment to find out what works best for you. Some people use an app, such as our new Livy Method app to record water, some use elastic bands on a water bottle, some fill a large container every day…More ideas will come up in the group discussions as we go.

7. **Do other drinks count towards water intake?**

Yes, all drinks except alcohol count towards water intake.

8. **Should I buy a water filter?**

This is a personal choice. Although it's always a good idea to make sure the water you are drinking is safe, it's up to you whether or not you want to use a filter.

9. **Can I have carbonated or sparkling water?**

It is fine on occasion, but you want the majority of your water intake to be flat water.

10. **I'm having trouble drinking so much water. Any tips?**

Start early in the day, set reminders on your phone with a goal of how much you want to drink each hour. Get a nice water bottle. Try using a straw. It will become easier as you go along.

11. **Why do I have dry lips and a pasty mouth even though I'm drinking tons of water?**

These can be signs that you are still not fully hydrated and the body is asking for more water, or it can be a sign you are going into detox, so try increasing water slightly. Keep in mind this can also be due to medications or underlying health issues.

LET'S TALK LOW SODIUM

Sodium is the main component of salt and an essential electrolyte which helps with balancing water in the body, muscle function and nerve transmissions.

For years, health organizations have been warning people about the dangers of salt, linking too much sodium to high blood pressure and recommending people limit their intake. However, even though too much sodium causes problems, consuming too little can be just as unhealthy.

Insufficient sodium in your blood can occur when water and sodium are out of balance. In other words, there's either too much water or not enough sodium in your blood. Symptoms of low blood sodium can vary from person to person and can cause serious issues if not addressed.

Common symptoms of low blood sodium include:

- weakness
- fatigue or low energy
- headache
- nausea
- vomiting
- muscle cramps or spasms
- confusion
- irritability

**As you can see, some of the same symptoms of low sodium are also similar to detox, so keep that in mind. **

Although it's worth noting, low sodium levels are few and far between. Unless you are excessively drinking way more water than you need, sweating excessively, taking medication that can cause low sodium issues or avoiding salt, chances are there is nothing for you to be concerned about.

Many factors can cause low blood sodium. Your sodium levels may get too low if your body loses too much water and electrolytes but may also be caused by certain medical conditions.

Including:

- severe vomiting or diarrhea.
- taking certain medications, including antidepressants and pain medications.
- taking diuretics (water pills).
- drinking too much water during exercise (this is very rare).
- dehydration (please note low sodium can also be due to not enough water).

- kidney disease or kidney failure.
- liver disease.
- heart problems, including congestive heart failure.
- adrenal gland disorders such as Addison's disease, which affects your adrenal gland's ability to regulate the balance of sodium, potassium, and water in your body.
- hypothyroidism (underactive thyroid).
- primary polydipsia, a condition in which excess thirst makes you drink too much.
- using ecstasy or other hard-core drugs.
- syndrome of inappropriate antidiuretic hormone (SIADH), which makes your body retain water.
- diabetes insipidus, a rare condition in which the body doesn't make antidiuretic hormones.
- Cushing's syndrome, which causes high cortisol levels (this is rare).

(Sourced from Healthline)

WHO NEEDS TO BE MINDFUL OF LOW SODIUM?

- People who are older in age
- People who use diuretics
- If you use antidepressants
- If you are sweating a lot due to climate or exercise
- If eating a low-sodium diet
- If you have had heart failure, kidney disease, or other conditions

If you have any of these risk factors for low sodium, you may need to be more careful about your intake of water and be sure to add in salt or trace minerals as needed.

A blood test can help your doctor check for low sodium levels.

TIPS FOR PREVENTING LOW SODIUM IN YOUR BLOOD:

- Keeping your water and electrolyte levels in balance can help prevent low blood sodium.
- Simply being sure to include sodium in your diet by salting foods with Pink Himalayan or sea salt, adding in the Sole Water (which we will talk about later), or adding in trace minerals to your water is not only healthy for you, but an easy way to ensure you are getting the sodium you need.

The moral of the story here:

- Be mindful of your water intake. Although water is key to the process, you want to be making sure you are drinking enough, and not just adding in more than you need. Be thoughtful when you are increasing water. If you are thirsty and in detox, listen to the body's cues and drink more when needed.

- You need salt in your diet, as much as you have been told it's bad for you...just like most things in the diet industry...that's a half truth. Be mindful of adding it in when following a healthy diet.

- If you have any concerns at all with your sodium levels, it is always recommended to get blood work done to confirm and to work with your health care professional.

LET'S TALK COFFEE

Coffee is totally fine to have on plan but here are a few things to note:

- You can drink as much coffee as you like but try to avoid drinking it later in the day if it messes with your sleep.

- Coffee counts towards your water intake, although it's not ideal so be sure not to use it as the main source.

- You can use any type of creamer you like, dairy or non dairy, but we suggest you avoid any artificial flavour or colour. So look for naturally flavoured and watch the amount of sugar added to some creamers.

- You can use real sugar, raw sugar or natural sweeteners like honey or maple syrup.

- I'm not a fan of agave. It is super sweet and high in fructose, which can feed into the need for something sweet and lead to insulin resistance, so best to avoid.

- And when it comes to artificial sweeteners, even though there are some better ones on the market like stevia and monk fruit, they can still lead to insulin resistance, so try to avoid it.

(Insulin resistance is when your body (pancreas) over produces insulin, something we will be focusing on further as we go...the goal is to decrease the amount your body needs to use).

LET'S TALK ALCOHOL

This is a hot topic when it comes to weight loss, so let's discuss how alcohol fits into the plan.

When it comes to weight loss, I've never had a client or group member have to stop drinking alcohol in order to lose weight. Generally, that's because alcohol is not the reason your body is feeling a need to store fat. With that said, there are benefits to limiting your intake so still be mindful of what you are drinking when looking to lose weight.

If you like to enjoy a beverage every now and then, following these tips can help minimize the impact on your body and the scale.

- Most important tip is to get extra water in to compensate for dehydration that alcohol can cause. We recommend a minimum extra cup (250 ml/8 oz) of water per drink.

WINE

- Choose red wine over white. Although both are fine, red has more antioxidants and is slightly better for you. That isn't a reason to give up your white if that's what you prefer.

ROSE & CHAMPAGNES

- A little higher in sugar so don't be surprised if you wake up with a headache but also totally fine to have.

BEER/CIDERS

- Avoid "light" or "low-cal" beer. Light beer may have less calories but turns to sugar faster. That is an issue because we are not worried about calories, we are more concerned about how it breaks down in the body and affects your insulin levels and digestive system. Darker beers like Guinness are higher in nutrient value but any of your regular, all-natural ales, lagers, pilsners etc. are totally fine.

HARD LIQUOR

- When it comes to the hard stuff, be mindful about what you are using as a mix. Try to avoid pop/soda, including diet and flavoured juice.
- Stick with carbonated water, mixed with a splash of natural juices, tomato juice or Clamato etc. If you enjoy something like rye and coke or gin and tonic once every now and then, it's no big deal.

The issue with alcohol is more the food you eat with it. If you are following the plan this is a non-issue but sometimes you might be at a party and be mindfully indulging. Here's a couple of things to keep in mind if you are.

- Drinking alcohol slows down the metabolism & your digestive system, so you want to avoid any heavy carbs like bread and pasta and stick to more protein, fats (like cheese and nuts) and veggies.

- Keep in mind alcohol can affect weight loss in other ways. For example, interrupting your sleep, messing with estrogen levels, causing dehydration, and causing you to crave both sugar and salt the next day. Alcohol increases the production of galanin, a neuropeptide in the brain, which causes you to crave greasy food. Pair that with the effects of dehydration that causes you to crave sugar and you are ready to eat your face off the next day!

- Bumping up good fats like oils, nuts, seeds, and avocados, increasing your water along with having a banana, which is high in potassium, first thing the next day will help the body metabolize the alcohol and reduce the galanin.

- Drinking can also affect the good bacteria in your digestive system, so if your stomach always feels off the next day, try adding in or doubling up on your probiotic. I will be talking more about probiotics and other supplements in the next few weeks.

MY FINAL TIP

The best thing you can do to offset negative effects of alcohol consumption is to add in that extra water of one cup per drink.

Besides that, enjoy your beverages!

Please take time to head over to the Facebook Group and watch the quick video that accompanies this post.

LET'S TALK SHIFT WORK

How to manage the food plan with around the clock and off hours.

First, it's key to know that having a crazy or busy work schedule is not going to hinder your progress.

Working shift work can throw off your body's natural circadian rhythm, which in turn can cause you to be extra tired.

When tired, the body looks for pick-me-ups like carbs, caffeine, and sugar. This is generally a sign the body is asking for more water. Making water your focus will not only help with your energy levels but will also eliminate any cravings which will help you stay on track.

The more routine you can be with the food and water the better.

TIPS FOR WORKING OUT AN EATING SCHEDULE:

The basic rule for shift workers when it comes to the food plan is to start your day from when you wake up, regardless of what time of day that might be.

Even if it's 3pm or 9pm, wake up and have your warm lemon water or ACV and then your higher protein breakfast.

If you are eating breakfast at 9pm you may be more inclined to have something like fish or chicken and veg as opposed to more "breakfast-y" type foods, and that's ok.

If your day is broken up by taking naps, you can just insert the naps in your day and stick to your regular scheduled plan for food.

FOR EXAMPLE:

If you get up at 9am but then go back to bed at 12pm, you can have breakfast and then fruit... then nap. Or just breakfast then nap, then fruit when you wake up. When you wake up, continue with your day where you left off food wise, so in this case, go straight to lunch, if you had fruit before, or the fruit if you didn't, and then continue on with your day.

You also can extend your eating times by breaking your lunch and/or dinner portion into 2 servings. If you are working and awake for extended hours, it could look something like this:

- Breakfast
- Fruit
- 1/2 of lunch
- Other 1/2 of lunch
- Veg snack

- Nut/seeds snack
- 1/2 dinner
- Other 1/2 of dinner

This will have you eating 8 times a day so you can cover more hours.

Once we add in bonus snacks, they will also help with planning your day. For now, try to follow the food plan formula as much as possible. Bonus snacks are extra snacks you add to your day that can help fill in the gaps for those who get up extra early, those of you who are more active, and those of you who work shift work and will be awake sometimes for 24hrs.

As you become more in-tune with your hunger levels, you will notice some days you will feel hungrier than others. When working the night shift, for example, you may find your appetite is much lighter compared to the day, which is normal.

It might take you a while to find the right balance, don't stress. Play around with the timing until you find what works.

I will revisit this again when we introduce bonus snacks next week. Hope this helps!

Please take time to head over to the Facebook Group and watch the quick video that accompanies this post and if you need help with planning around your shifts, be sure to ask.

LET'S TALK THE SCALE

Let's take a moment and talk about the Scale.

I know many of you are not fans of stepping on the scale every day and for some of you it can be downright frustrating. Which is why it is ultimately up to you if you are going to use it while following the Program.

During weight loss the scale acts as a tool. Personally, I feel it can be very insightful, which is why I suggest you step on the scale every day during this process.

Trying to lose weight without using a scale is like trying to build a house without a hammer. It can be done…but it is so much easier when you use the right tools.

The scale can help indicate where your body is at in the process based on how it's responding in combination with the foods you are eating, the water you are drinking, and the supplements you are taking… along with how you are feeling from day to day.

HERE IS HOW TO USE IT SO YOU CAN LOSE IT!

What's happening on the scale can help you stay on top of the changes your body is making day to day and help you make the adjustments that help speed up the fat loss process and help the body focus on letting go of the fat.

Here are a couple rules about weight loss and weight gain that are helpful to understand before you let the scale freak you out or frustrate you.

When it comes to the scale, using My Method, a drop is always a drop. When the scale moves down, you can count on it being because of actual fat loss and that is your true weight. Whereas when the scale is up, it is always a superficial gain based on what you did or didn't eat or drink the day before.

So, when you say, "I gained weight last night" or "Why is my weight up even though I'm doing everything right?!" understand that it's impossible for your body to take the foods you eat and convert them into fat overnight. It's harder and takes longer than you think for your body to make fat.

- It is key to understand that weight loss is based on momentum, NOT on how you ate the day before.
- Meaning, weight loss happens after your body has geared up to go into "weight loss mode" which can be days or even a week.
- "Weight loss mode", or in "detox mode" are the loose and very general terms I use to describe when the body is specifically focused on fat loss.

THINGS TO KEEP IN MIND:

The scale is going to fluctuate. It will go up and down and you will have plateaus. Real weight loss is not a straight line down. Fluctuations are normal and expected.

- It is normal when you drop fat to have your weight go down on the scale & then back up again as fat cells retain water before they have time to shrink…it does not mean you gained weight back.

- It's also normal to feel bloated and gross and have your weight up the day before it shows a drop on the scale…. this is not real weight gain, it's a sign to stay on plan because your weight is about to drop.

- It is also normal to feel like you have lost weight, but the scale is showing the same number or is up. This is usually a sign you are about to drop it just hasn't translated on the scale yet.

- Drinking your water is so important! Water helps to get your body into detox, so it drops the fat in the first place. Not drinking enough water can slow the process of seeing the scale move.

- If the scale is bouncing up and down, it usually means your body needs more water because it is trying to get into detox.

OTHER THINGS TO KEEP IN MIND:

- Best time to weigh yourself is in the morning after you go to the bathroom.

- A digital scale is ideal as you can see the small fluctuations, which can be helpful.

- The body doesn't care about how much you want the scale to move. It has no concept of time or your desire to lose weight as fast as possible.

- Your body also has no concept of any number you want to reach on the scale. Which is why going by how you feel can be just as important as stepping on the scale.

LET'S TALK ABOUT GOAL WEIGHT:

What is a good weight for you?

Without sounding cliché, I really do think it's when you feel comfortable in your skin. A good base line I use for clients is your lowest weight after the age of 21, that you were able to easily maintain.

That doesn't mean if you have always carried extra weight that you can't weigh less than you ever have, because you totally can. I always say weight loss is a side effect of being healthy. A properly functioning body has no need for excess fat, so given the opportunity and the time, it will be more than happy to get rid of it.

It is good to set a target weight as a goal, but I find most people underestimate their goals out of fear of failing. Group members are always setting new goals along the way and that's ok because it's a process.

On a final note, I have attached some photos (refer to the original group post) as a visual for you to see what weight loss really looks like on the scale. It is not the typical straight line down most believe it to be. It is very normal for weight to go up and down and up and down and be perceived to be all over the place when there actually is a pattern to it.

TO RECAP:

- As frustrating as it can be sometimes, the scale is a very helpful tool for weight loss and nothing to be feared.

- Best time to weigh yourself is first thing in the morning, ideally after going to the bathroom. Later in the day the scale will always read higher.

- Your weight being up does not mean you gained weight. It is normal for your weight to fluctuate whether you are losing weight or not for a variety of reasons.

- A new low on the scale is always real weight loss and is your actual weight.

- It's also normal to feel bloated and gross and have your weight up the day before it shows a drop on scale.

- It's normal to "feel like" you have lost weight but have the scale up or the same. This also can be a sign you are about to drop.

- Weight loss is never a straight line down. The scale is going to go up and down whether you like it or not. It's a normal part of the process and is natural for the body even after you have finished losing weight.

I will be talking more in-depth about your body's response to the process and how to use the scale to your advantage as we move forward.

Please take time to head over to the Facebook Group to review the visuals and watch the quick video that accompanies this post.

LET'S TALK TO THE MEN

It may seem like there are not a lot of men in the group but there are!

It's just that women tend to be more vocal about weight loss and the process.

Things to keep in mind for the guys:

- There is nothing men need to do differently.

- Follow the plan as designed and it will work wonders for both men & women.

- Eat all meals and snacks.

- Make your food as nutrient rich as possible and don't be afraid to add in the heavier carbs as needed.

- Eat to satisfaction and don't try to eat less.

- Get the water in!

Men tend to lose weight a lot faster than women, which can be an issue. With that said, It's a good issue to have, but one to be mindful of. Because the body can make change fast, it is a good idea to be checking in with your health care provider along the way. Especially if you have any health issues or are taking any medication.

As we progress, I will be addressing the men in the group specifically and will be sure to let you know if there are any tweaks or changes you need to make along the way.

Please take time to head over to the Facebook Group and watch the quick video that accompanies this post.

LET'S TALK DETOX

How we use the body's natural detox process to lose weight.

**"Detox" is a loose term I use to describe when the body is specifically focused on fat loss or in what I call "weight loss mode". **

It is key to note the body doesn't need any help when it comes to detoxing naturally. This is why I'm not a fan of detox kits, detox juice, or juice cleanses. When it comes to detox and helping the body get the fat out, there is nothing you need to do other than follow the program.

The program is systematically designed to do all the work for you. There is nothing you need to do other than follow it exactly as designed.

Keep in mind not everyone will experience detox symptoms. If you don't experience symptoms that doesn't mean you aren't going into detox, everyone is different. You can be just as successful on plan without experiencing typical detox symptoms as someone who experiences strong detox symptoms.

Some typical "detox" symptoms include:

- feeling rundown
- flu-like symptoms
- runny nose
- dizzy as hormones balance
- headaches, chills, night sweats, aches and pains (nothing severe)
- feeling tired
- feeling bloated
- metallic taste in your mouth
- being thirsty and having dry lips even though you are drinking lots of water
- waking up around 3-4am to pee
- loose bowel movements and/or constipation
- Itchy skin or mild rashes (nothing severe)

Although some of you may experience strong detox symptoms, there is no need for concern. There is nothing you will do on this program that will cause, or lead to, any detrimental effects in the body.

**If you feel something is off, please make sure to always check in with your health care provider with any concerns. **

Keep in mind, all you are doing is eating healthy food and drinking enough water to be hydrated. It's the changes in food, the design of the food plan formula, and the process of getting the fat out that causes the body to react. You can't expect your body to make life changing changes without noticing.

With that said, it's amazing what the body can do and how it will respond when you are giving it what it needs.

Please take time to head over to the Facebook Group and watch the quick video that accompanies this post.

PROTEINS, CARBS, AND FATS

In my Program I talk a lot about the mix of protein, carbs, and fats that your body needs. And while this isn't something I need you to think too much about, here is a brief outline for those interested.

PLEASE NOTE: you do NOT need to worry about percentages or portions. Serving size and portion wise, all you need to do right now is follow the plan and eat to satisfaction.

This is just to give you examples of what foods fall under each category.

SOURCES OF CARBS (foods that break down into energy)

- Fruit

- Vegetables

- Heavier Root Veg like potatoes, squash, cassava, plantain

- Naturally occurring sugar found in things like beans and lentils and chickpeas

- Oatmeal and cereal like hemp hearts and buckwheat

- Rice and grains like black rice & quinoa, barley

- Ryvita crackers and Ezekiel bread

SOURCES OF PROTEIN (feeds the muscles helping to repair and rebuild along with maintain and build muscle mass)

- Fish

- Meat (Any Meat)

- Eggs

- Seafood

- Beans, lentils, legumes

- Nuts and Seeds

- Incomplete protein like oatmeal, quinoa and rice (not to be used as main source)

- Dairy cheese, yogurt, milk products (not to be used as a main source)

- Tofu

PLANT PROTEIN

As you can see below, there is protein found in lots of things besides animal sources.

- Broccoli 2.6g per 1 cup

- Asparagus 2.4g per 1 cup

- Peas 9g per 1 cup

- Cauliflower 2g per 1 cup

- Brussels 3g per 1 cup

- Bok choy 1g per 1 cup

- Spinach, collard greens 1g per 1 cup

- Mung bean sprouts 2.5g per 1 cup

- Beans (kidney, pinto, black beans, chick peas etc.) 7.5g per 1/2 cup

- Lentils 9g per 1/2 cup

- Quinoa 4g per 1/2 cup

- Tempeh 11g per 1/2 cup

- Tofu 7g per 1/2 cup

- Buckwheat 6g per 1 cup

- Soy beans/Edamame 10g per 1/2 cup

- Rice 7g per 1cup

- Hemp seeds 10g per 3 tbsp

- Pumpkin seeds 5g per oz

- Chia 4g per 2 tbsp

- Nut butter -15g per 2 tbsp

- Ezekiel bread 8g per 2 slices

- Hummus 7g per 2 tbsp

- Spirulina 4g per 1 tbsp

Keep in mind you DO NOT need to worry about these measurements.

They are for reference only and to point out the fact that some proteins have carbs in them, some vegetables have protein in them, and that protein adds up.

As long as you are following the plan as outlined, you are getting enough and the right mix of everything you need.

SOURCES OF FATS (essential for cellular function, providing alternative energy and brain fuel)

- Fish/Fish oil

- Omega 3 and or 369

- Alternative oils like olive oil, coconut oil, avocado oil, grape seed oil, flax and hemp oil
- Salad dressings with good quality oils
- Olives
- Avocado
- Nuts
- Seeds
- Hemp hearts
- Dairy...like yogurt, cheese, butter

This is not a complete list, it is just to give you an idea of the kind of foods I'm suggesting when talking about incorporating proteins, carbs and fats to your meals.

Please take time to head over to the Facebook Group and watch the quick video that accompanies this post.

LET'S TALK CONDIMENTS

This is a quick one, pretty much all condiments are fine to use. What you want to look for is quality ingredients, so nothing artificial.

Avoid:

- Artificial flavour
- Artificial colour
- Hydrogenated oil

Follow that rule and you should be fine.

This is for sauces and gravies and dips and all condiments in general. Use at will to flavour your foods.

Now, with that said some condiments can be super salty and may lead to the scale being up the next day...soy sauce is one of the main ones that has that effect. It is nothing to worry about and not a reason to not use it, as it's not real weight gain… just key to note when weighing yourself.

Please take time to head over to the Facebook Group and watch the quick video that accompanies this post.

LET'S TALK DAIRY

Now if you are not into dairy, that's cool...you don't need to eat it or add it in. We get a lot of questions about dairy on plan so hopefully this post will help break things down for you!

FIRST LET'S TALK ABOUT CHEESE

WHEN CAN I HAVE IT?

- With any of your meals AND it can also be added to your veg snack. With the veg snack just make sure raw veggies are the star of the show.

HOW MUCH CAN I HAVE?

- As with all meals and snacks on plan you are to eat to satisfaction...so add cheese to your meal and then eat said meal to satisfaction. See below regarding concerns about cholesterol.

WHAT KINDS OF CHEESE CAN I HAVE?

- Pretty much any kind is fine, avoid any processed cheese and of course any cheese with anything artificial in it including artificial colours.

- White cheeses are great, especially old white cheddar.

- Processed cheeses include things like Velveeta, Cheese Whiz, American Cheese, Kraft Cheese Slices, Cheese Strings, any cheese that comes in a tube or jar. Pre-shredded cheese has some questionable anti-caking agents so it is fine to have occasionally but keep it to a minimum.

- Always look for all natural ingredients.

- Avoid "light" or low-fat cheeses as they often contain additives to compensate for the fat removed.

WHAT IF I'M CONCERNED ABOUT CHOLESTEROL?

- When it comes to avoiding high cholesterol, it's all about the kind of fats you are consuming.

- Cheese is a saturated fat and you do need to be mindful about how much saturated fat you consume.

- Saturated fat is a good fat, BUT the key is to make sure you are getting enough great fat like omega 3 and omega 6.

- If you are following the plan, this isn't something you need to worry about as the plan factors it in. Just be sure to be adding a mix of good fat to your meals.

To review a list of good fats, check out the post on Proteins, Carbs & Fats.

LET'S TALK ABOUT YOGURT

WHEN CAN I HAVE IT?

For the first part of the program yogurt is eaten mostly at breakfast with added protein such as **hemp hearts, nuts, seeds, nut butters and/or protein powder.**

It can also be added to lunch and dinner as an added dip, dressing, sauce, or condiment to your meal. It can also be used as a dip with your afternoon veg. snack.

WHAT KINDS CAN I HAVE?

Plain, Greek yogurt is the best option as it is higher in protein and lower in carbs. This is because of the straining process used to make it. By removing the excess liquid whey and lactose (natural sugars) a higher protein yogurt is created!

Avoid low or no-fat yogurts because they usually contain additives to compensate for the lack of fat that can jack up the carbs and sugars. There are some low & no-fat Greek yogurts that don't contain any additives, but we want the fat and protein for more sustaining energy, especially at breakfast.

CAN I HAVE FLAVOURED OR SWEETENED YOGURT?

Yes, you can but make sure it has a higher fat content to neutralize the amount of insulin needed to break it down. Again, look for Greek yogurts higher in fat (4%+) and always bump it up even more with the above-mentioned proteins. The more sugar, the more fat and protein needed.

A better alternative to sweetened yogurt is to use plain and add a touch of honey or maple syrup instead. Or mix your favourite sweetened yogurt with plain yogurt. That way you have control over the amount of sugar added and can slowly reduce it as your taste buds adjust.

WHAT ABOUT NON-DAIRY OR PLANT-BASED YOGURTS?

Same guidelines apply. Look for higher protein and fat without any artificial ingredients. Always add in extra protein as mentioned above.

LET'S TALK ABOUT MILK AND CREAM

WHEN CAN I HAVE IT?

Milk and cream can be used at any time. You can have a glass of milk whenever you like, and it would count towards your water/fluid intake. Milk and cream can also be added to coffee, tea, high protein cereals, oatmeal, soups, sauces etc. at will.

WHAT KINDS CAN I HAVE?

When it comes to milk and dairy you don't have to avoid low or no fat. The removal of fat here doesn't require additives to compensate for taste or texture. The fat is simply removed. So, you can enjoy anything from skim to full fat when it comes to milk and cream.

WHAT ABOUT LACTOSE FREE AND PLANT-BASED MILKS AND FLAVOURED CREAMERS?

Those are all fine to have on plan. When it comes to flavoured creamers, whether they are dairy or non-dairy, just make sure they are made with all natural ingredients, nothing artificial, and watch the amount of sugar added as some can be very high.

Keep in mind that although all dairy products have protein, they aren't a good "stand-alone" protein on program so should always be used in addition to other protein sources when eaten with meals. Check out the Grocery List for other protein sources.

Please take time to head over to the Facebook Group and watch the quick video that accompanies this post.

LET'S TALK LEAFY GREENS

Leafy greens are an ideal addition to meals as they help to increase the Glucagon-like-Peptide-1 hormone that keeps blood sugar more stable and helps keep you more satisfied. They are also packed with tons of nutrients that are great for your health and cellular function and an excellent source of fiber which helps the body process food through your digestive system, which is needed for weight loss.

Plus, all of the changes you are making in your diet can affect your bowel movements. Leafy greens provide the roughage your body needs to keep you regular.

Leafy greens can be added to meals raw, like in a salad, but also cooked or sautéed and/or added to soups, stews & stir fries. Cabbage, Brussels sprouts, and bok choy, among others which are listed in the Grocery List, are also classified as veg and can be used as one or the other or both in your meals.

The general rule is...if it's green and leafy it works!

Getting your leafy greens in can be difficult especially in the colder months but cooking them and adding them to soups, stews etc. is a great way to get them in when you're not feeling like a salad.

If you are not a fan of eating your leafy greens, it is still key to get them in. You don't have to be fancy about it or get in a huge variety. It's also not a big deal if you are a bit hit and miss getting them in, as long as you are mindful to be as consistent as possible.

Although they are suggested at lunch and dinner, leafy greens can also be added to breakfast or the raw veg snack.

Please take time to head over to the Facebook Group and watch the quick video that accompanies this post.

LUNCH AND DINNER VISUAL GUIDELINE

Don't Take This Too Literally. I can't stress it enough. It's only meant as a visual guideline. We don't want you to start dividing up your plate.

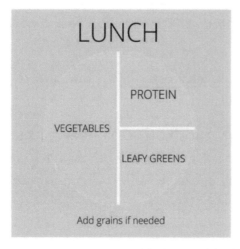
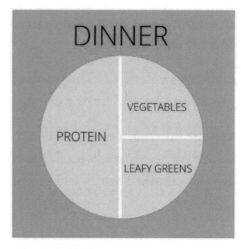

ADD HEALTHY FATS AT WILL

Sometimes at lunch, your protein portion may be a bit bigger, or at dinner a bit smaller. Sometimes you may only have a pinch of greens added to a soup etc. As long as you just keep the focus on veg at lunch and protein at dinner you are totally fine. Even if it's totally off balance sometimes, it's no big deal! The point is to have you start thinking more about what you are eating and getting in some nicely balanced meals.

NOTHING NEEDS TO BE EXACT AND, WHATEVER YOU DO, DON'T MEASURE!

Sometimes you might be eating a chili, stew, soup or stir fry where the divided plate doesn't apply. As long as there is a good balance of veggies and protein you are good. When in doubt, toss in a bit of extra protein or veg if you feel the need. We just want you to start paying attention.

Portions Eat to satisfaction. This looks different for everyone. We would rather you be overeating right now rather than undereating, so do not try to cut your portions. This will make more sense as we move forward.

Most importantly try not to overthink it. If your meals are slightly off balance, it's not going to affect your progress. If you are eating nutrient rich, whole foods, and following the guidelines, you are right on track!

Note About "Grains as Needed" This will become easier to gauge as we move along but basically if you are feeling you need a little more "oomph" to your meal, add them in. Like you are looking at your nice clean salad and thinking "I don't think this is going to satisfy me today" then add some grains or heavier carb veggies like potatoes etc.

LET'S TALK ABOUT GUM

Can you chew it on Plan?

It is not advised and here is why:

Digestion starts in the mouth, technically with smell first and then by chewing. Chewing gum artificially stimulates your digestive system, and without following through and eating food, that can be an issue. Especially if the gum you are chewing is artificially flavored and made with artificial sweetener.

Some sweeteners like sucralose, although low in sugar and calories, still causes a reaction in the body that secretes insulin (the chemical your body uses after it breaks down food to convert glucose into energy).

In small amounts it's a minimal concern, but if you chew a lot of gum it can lead to insulin resistance and higher insulin levels that can signal weight gain. We are trying to reduce the amount of insulin your body is used to using, which is why I suggest minimizing any gum chewing.

IF YOU NEED TO CHEW:

Try to chew natural gum, these can be found online or at health food stores. Try to chew directly after a meal as opposed to in between.

Avoid using it to suppress your appetite, you want to be in-tune to your body's needs not suppress them. In no way is chewing gum a benefit.

NOTE: MINTS HAVE THE SAME EFFECT

Please take time to head over to the Facebook Group and watch the quick video that accompanies this post.

LET'S TALK CHOCOLATE

Dark chocolate can be a source of magnesium and, when it's good quality, it can be low in sugar. So, can you have it on plan?

I'm going to say NO and here's why:

You don't want to be using food for anything other than nutritional requirements right now. The goal is to get in tune to your body's needs and cut through your "wants". If you are craving sugar you want to ask yourself why? As every craving is a message from your body.

You don't want to be feeding into cravings or trying to manage or mask them. You want to address them, so you don't have them anymore. As always, when all is said and done, it's no big deal. It all depends on how much you want to get out of this process.

Down the road you will be able to add chocolate back in, but for now, if you are looking to maximize your results, I suggest keeping it out. If you are concerned about sugar cravings, then simply follow the plan. As the Program is designed to address them.

Eat all of your meals and snacks, make your food nutrient rich, eat to satisfaction, and drink your water. With that said, nothing is make or break and no one is expecting perfection. If you do end up eating some chocolate or indulging in any treats, all you need to do is keep moving forward and get back at it.

Please take time to head over to the Facebook Group and watch the quick video that accompanies this post.

LET'S TALK ABOUT EXERCISE

How to incorporate it into the Program and tweak it so it is more conducive to fat loss.

As you move through The Program and focus more and more on giving the body what it needs, it will start to allow you more access to your energy reserves by maximizing your metabolism. Your metabolism is the rate at which your body functions day to day or to simplify, how much energy you use and calories you naturally burn on a daily basis.

When the body feels a need to store fat, it will keep you in "reserve mode" and limit the amount of energy you can use. This is why mentally you might be keen to exercise but energetically you might not feel so motivated.

As you move forward in this process and continue to put the time and energy into giving your body what it needs, your body is going to start giving you access to more energy. After a few weeks on the program, you may be surprised that you will want to move your body more and feel like being more active.

Although there are many beneficial reasons to exercise, it is not a mandatory requirement for weight loss on this program.

We will however be talking more about it as we move forward for those interested.

AMPLIFYING YOUR FITNESS FOR FAT LOSS:

Let's talk about the best way to implement exercises that will fall in line with your weight loss goals: If you are new to exercise, I suggest you start by simply being more active.

I know it sounds cliché, but things like taking the stairs and parking further away when getting groceries, going for walks or doing some push-ups or squats in your kitchen, can add up and have a big impact.

If you are looking for something more intense, there are a lot of great home workout options. It's best to start slow to minimize the stress on the body and build up to it. Whatever you choose to do, it should be something you enjoy so you make a positive association to exercise moving forward and it becomes something you look forward to doing.

**You also want to walk away from any exercise feeling good and energized, not tired, taxed or drained. **

You have to remember that you are working towards getting the body to focus on detox and fat loss. If you work out too hard and you create too much damage in the body, it will have no choice but to focus on repairing and rebuilding instead of detoxing and fat loss.

THIS BRINGS US TO THE TOPIC OF REST:

If you are going to work out to the point of being sore, you need to make sure you are giving your body adequate time to repair and rebuild, or you will run the risk of overtraining.

Overtraining happens when the body can't catch up to the damage that's been done, leaving your body feeling weak and in a deficit. Which in turn can cause the body to feel the need to hold on to fat or store more fat for easy energy.

LET'S TALK CARDIO OR GETTING YOUR HEART RATE UP:

When it comes to exercise and weight loss, it's all about the message you are sending to the body. Your physical brain that runs your body doesn't see what you are doing for exercise, it only interprets what you are doing based on your movements and heart rate. This is where you can use the body's natural FIGHT or FLIGHT response to maximize your results.

Getting your heart rate up as high as you can for as long as you can, even if just for a few minutes, evokes the FIGHT or FLIGHT response in the body and immediately sends a message for the body to boost your metabolism and work to make you stronger.

The body's sole responsibility is to keep you alive, so if you repeatedly evoke the fight or flight response, your body will look to make you as strong and efficient as possible. In wanting to be as efficient as possible, your body will look to get rid of any extra fat that could be slowing you down. This makes cardio (exercise that gets your heart rate up) very effective for fat loss.

Cardio doesn't have to be running, it can be walking fast, skipping, swimming, dancing, lifting lighter weights with higher reps, sports activities, and anything else that helps get your heart rate up.

With cardio you are basically taking the muscle you already have in your body and using it to move your body, which will get your heart rate up without creating damage, making it a complement to the weight loss program.

LET'S TALK LIFTING WEIGHTS:

When it comes to lifting weights, things can get tricky because you are purposely creating damage in the body, so the body repairs the damage and makes the muscle stronger.

That is great for bone density, building muscle and shaping your body, but not great for fat loss. That doesn't mean you can't continue to lift weights, especially if that is something you enjoy. I would, however, suggest you lift a little lighter using higher repetitions, to use the muscle you do have to help to get your heart rate up with minimal damage.

During sleep is when the body detoxes and/or makes change, it doesn't do both at the same time. So, if your body is always sore, then your body is always focusing on repairing the damage that is making you sore. Leaving very little or no time left to focus on detox.

I know we have been taught to believe that exercise is how you lose weight. But that just isn't true. In fact, exercise is a really crappy weight loss tool and can actually work against you when it comes to the scale.

Now with that said, exercise is amazing for so many reasons, like stress release, heart health, and making your body stronger in general, so I'm not saying don't do it. I'm just saying be smart about it and understand the message that is being sent to the body when you do.

MY EXERCISE FAVES FOR FAT LOSS:

- Walking because it's also conducive to healing and the least stressful type of exercise you can do.
- Anything outside, because it stimulates the brain and works the body while communing with nature and relieving stress.
- Dance or Boxing/Martial arts type classes that move the body in different ways other than side to side and up and down, while evoking the fight response.
- Biking or spinning is great for getting your heart rate up and evoking the flight response.
- Exercises that use your own body weight as resistance.

Let me know if you have any questions and be sure to check with your doctor before starting, or if for any reason you are feeling apprehensive about adding exercise into your routine.

Please take time to head over to the Facebook Group and watch the quick video that accompanies this post.

LET'S TALK BREAD, FLOURS, PASTA, AND CRACKERS

We're mindful of not giving people the impression that this program is low Carb...because it's not. It's more about the right carbs. On plan you are eating veggies and fruit, grains and legumes, with naturally occurring sugars...so the plan, if followed, is far from low carb.

We get asked a lot if it's okay to eat bread, pasta, crackers etc. on plan. The answer is yes, BUT...

By following the Food Plan you are trying to decrease the amount of insulin your body is used to using. Which in turn will help you to feel more satisfied with smaller portions.

Bread, pasta, and flour in general, require a lot more insulin than whole foods when the body breaks them down, regardless of the type or source. So, when it comes to weight loss and this process, we consider bread and pasta to be processed foods. You can eat them, BUT it can slow down the process.

BREAD & CRACKERS

Although it is possible to lose weight on this program while continuing to eat bread it can slow down the process. In the beginning we want you to have an easy transition into following the food plan so it's okay to keep bread in and keep it with breakfast or lunch, but not both.

It's also important the type of bread you choose. Best choice is Ezekiel Bread which is a high quality, sprouted grain bread that doesn't contain any flour. Because it is free from any preservatives and sugar it is found in the fridge or freezer section in health food stores and many grocery stores.

Ezekiel Bread ingredient list: *Organic Sprouted Wheat, Filtered Water, Organic Sprouted Barley, Organic Sprouted Millet, Organic Malted Barley, Organic Sprouted Lentils, Organic Sprouted Soybeans, Organic Sprouted Spelt, Fresh Yeast, Organic Wheat Gluten, Sea Salt.*

If you can't find Ezekiel, and choose to keep bread in your diet, look for other sprouted grain breads that are dense, grainy, and seedy. Go for high fiber and quality ingredients. The less processed and shorter the ingredient list the better!

When it comes to crackers, we recommend high fibre crackers like Ryvita brand. Ryvita crackers have a short ingredient list, contain whole grains, and are high in fiber. If you can't find the Ryvita brand specifically, look for crackers with similar ingredients.

Ryvita Multi-Grain Crispbread Ingredients:

Whole grain rye flour, Toasted grains and seeds (buckwheat, soy meal, sesame seeds, flaxseed, kibbled rye), Rye bran, Salt.

Mary's Super Seed Crackers are a good gluten free alternative for those of you who can't digest gluten.

PASTA & FLOUR

We get asked a lot if it's okay to have pasta made with alternative flours such as chickpea, black bean or konjak. Although these pastas are a better choice than ones made with wheat flour, while trying to lose weight, it is recommended to leave them out.

It's not about what the pasta (or flour) is made from, it's about the process of making them that can still affect blood sugar levels. Right now, while trying to lose weight, we are working hard to decrease and balance out blood sugar levels so adding in pastas and larger quantities of flour is counterproductive.

Small amounts of flour used for breading or thickening a soup or sauce is totally fine as a small quantity won't have the same effect on your blood sugar levels.

As mentioned above, some people can continue to eat these things and still lose weight but if you are looking to Maximize your efforts you might want to consider limiting or skipping them altogether. Remember it's not a "lifestyle" it's an effort to lose as much weight as possible in the time frame we have. Maybe you prefer to take a more relaxed approach and leave it in. That's also totally cool! The choice is yours based on how hard core you want to be about the process.

We understand that bread and pasta are convenient, easy, and taste great and we know you might miss having them .... but you won't miss the fat when it's gone and keeping them out can make that fat loss process happen a lot faster.

MUST WATCH VIDEOS (FACEBOOK GROUP)

Before you move ahead with The Program, you must watch these 3 videos, which are posted in the Facebook Group, if you have not yet watched them.

MY METHOD:

- I explain why My Method is different from any other diet you have done. It is important you understand the method behind the process you will be following over the next 12 weeks.

THE FOOD PLAN:

- This is where I explain the rhyme and the reason behind what I'm asking you to eat and when, on the Food Plan. The sooner you start being consistent with the Food Plan, the sooner you will start and feel results.

DETOX VIDEO:

- This is where I explain how we use the body's natural detox process to help get fat out. It's key to understand how your body may or may not respond while following the Program.

As we go, I'll be talking more in depth about the Program and the Process. For now, focus on being consistent with the basics.

Please take time to head over to the Facebook Group and watch the quick videos that accompany this post.

WEEK 1 GUIDELINES: IMPLEMENTING THE FOOD PLAN

The goal is to implement the changes with the food if you haven't yet. And if you have, continue with the food plan, focus on water, be as consistent as possible, and pay attention to how your body is responding to the changes you are making.

Any information not included in the Workbook, including all of the accompanying videos, you will find in the Facebook Support Group. Everything is posted in the GUIDES section, where the GUIDES are listed by day for Days 1-7 and moving forward, they will be listed by the Week.

Another way to quickly find information in the Facebook Support Group is by using TOPICS, which is located on the same menu bar as GUIDES (mobile) or on the right-hand side of the page on a computer. You can also search for information by using the search feature located at the very top of the page.

Each day, we post additional support info/videos to further explain the process and any changes you are to make. These posts are not emailed out so be sure to check in to the Facebook Support Group every day.

THE GOAL FOR WEEK 1:

The goal for this first official week is to continue to implement the food plan, work on getting in the water, and be as consistent as possible. Also, if you need, take time to catch up on the information that has been posted and get yourself familiar with navigating the Group so you are up to date. We want to ensure you don't miss any need-to-know info moving forward.

MUST WATCH: If you have not seen them yet, please take the time to watch these videos (found in the Facebook Support Group) as they explain the basics of the program and the process.

- My Method
- The Food Plan
- Detox

THE FOCUS FOR THIS WEEK:

- Continue to follow the Food Plan Formula.
- Eat ALL meals and snacks.
- Make food choices as nutrient rich as possible.
- Eat to satisfaction, meaning do NOT try to eat less.
- Continue to work on getting your water in.
- Even though these are healthy changes you are making, change is stressful on the body, so consistency is key as you give it time to adjust.

Keep in mind, how you eat in the beginning will change and evolve week by week, and each week leads into and sets up the following week.

YOUR DAILY CHECKLIST:

- Check into the Facebook Support Group daily.
- Watch the "Daily Check in" video.
- Watch or read any new support posts.
- Ask any questions you have on the Questions of the Day Post, so you are clear on the changes you are making week to week.
- Implement the changes you need to make.

FACEBOOK LIVES:

The live Q&A Facebook Times:

- Monday to Friday 9 am EST
- Monday to Thursday 7 pm EST
- Saturdays 10 am EST.

If you are having trouble finding the Lives, here are some tips:

- Once you see a live, be sure to set notifications. You will be prompted to do this while watching for the first time.
- Depending on what kind of device you are using, look for a menu option that is "Media" "Videos" or "Photos". Check in those menus after refreshing your page. Once you figure out the quickest way to find the video on the device you are using, this will be easy.

***Please Note: Facebook Lives are NOT a mandatory part of the Program. You DO NOT need to watch them to be successful. ***

A LOOK AHEAD AT WEEK 2:
- The goal for Week 2 will be to fine tune and perfect the changes you have already made.
- We will also be introducing bonus snacks.
- We will also be talking about supplements and going over any that might be a benefit to the process moving forward.

Consistency is a super important part of this process as the first few weeks are all about giving the body what it needs so it no longer feels the need to store fat. The next step is to get the body to focus on detox and help it stay in detox long enough to drop the fat, so the more consistent you can be, the quicker you will start seeing results.

As you can see, it's a process. This may be a different process than you have experienced before but rest assured, it is a process that works and works well.

We are not concerned at all about anyone's ability to lose weight. The Program is all about following the plan, implementing the changes week to week, all while problem solving and moving forward.

Although this is a Weight Loss Program, the focus is NOT on the scale right now. It is NOT about how strong you start; it's about following through and finishing strong.

There will come a time where the scale will become the focus and main topic of conversation, but we are not there yet.

For now, focus on the basics and be as consistent as possible. It's the quickest way to get the scale moving and to keep it moving.

We have a long way to go, but there's no reason we can't have fun along the way. So, let's do this!

Please take time to head over to the Facebook Group and watch the quick video that accompanies this post.

LET'S TALK BREAKFAST

If you need to eat it & how high protein it needs to be.

Breakfast is not the most important meal of the day; however, it can be very beneficial to your day and this process.

When you wake up, you are already full of energy. So, you don't need to eat breakfast to get energy. That's why you have the option of skipping it, carrying on with your day, then going straight to your morning fruit snack. With that said though, there is absolutely a benefit to eating it.

Starting your day with a high protein breakfast is a great way to "break the fast" and get your body working harder from the get go. It pains me to say it, but that means burning more calories throughout your day! (And no, we still don't count calories.).

Going higher protein feeds the muscles without the need for as much insulin as carbs. High insulin levels signal weight gain in the body and we are trying to lower the amount of insulin your body uses on plan.

It's best to think about how you can maximize your meals and get the most bang for your buck portion wise, rather than trying to skew your meals to be something you enjoy. Meaning, be mindful not to be looking for variety, something to fit into your lifestyle ongoing, or to get excitement from your meals.

There will be lots of time for that later as we will be adding recipe share pages to the Facebook group. For now, make sure to review the post on Meal Ideas in the Facebook Group where we break down options and provide links to some amazing on-plan recipes!

The focus right now is to keep it simple and make sure to have the components you need at each meal and snack.

Ideally, you want to eat breakfast within 2.5 hours of waking. However, this is not a hard and fast rule. If you wake up at 5am and you are not active or exercising, you can still eat breakfast as late as 8-9 am and be fine. Some people are up earlier and some sleep later, and that might change day to day.

If you get up later, that gives you less time to eat breakfast before you need a snack, so you might skip breakfast and go straight to the fruit snack. We will be adding in bonus snacks to help fill in the blanks for those of you who are up early, are more active, or do shift work.

For now, play around with the timing of breakfast and then your fruit snack.

Please take time to head over to the Facebook Group and watch the quick video that accompanies this post.

LET'S TALK FRUIT SNACK

Why you need to have it and why you can't add anything with it.

Normally, it is a good idea to combine your carbs with a protein and fat, which can help neutralize the amount of insulin needed to break down your food.

Which may have you confused and wondering why are we eating the fruit on its own?! And why am I so adamant about that?

Regardless if you choose to skip breakfast or go higher protein...by mid-morning, your glycogen (energy) reserves are starting to deplete. The goal is to replenish those energy stores before the body has to dip into and utilize your emergency fat reserves.

Using your fat reserves sends a message to the body that you need your fat...so that is something we are ultimately trying to avoid.

When it comes to what fruit is best, that's up to you...no fruit is off limits, and you can choose to mix and match if you like.

Bananas, which we always get asked about, are a little higher in sugar but a great addition for anyone who may be more active or in need of potassium due to cramps while sleeping.

Please take time to head over to the Facebook Group and watch the quick video that accompanies this post.

LET'S TALK LUNCH

Why it's not all about having salads every day.

Think of VEGGIES as being the star of the show and build your lunch around them, following the guidelines of vegetables, protein, greens and grains if needed.

It's not all about salads, in fact it's key to note, the body doesn't tend to be as interested in salads in the cooler months as it is in the warmer months. Soups and stews along with foods like heavier carbs and fatty meats that create heat when you eat them are much more appealing.

Right now, with the time of year, if you do find salads appealing, be sure to load them up and make your lunch as nutrient rich as possible. Be sure to eat to satisfaction and be mindful that hunger levels change day to day.

Cheese, condiments, dressings, sauces, gravy and spices are all fine to use on plan. Best to leave out bread at lunch, as well as any kind of pasta and noodles.

Please take time to head over to the Facebook Group and watch the quick video that accompanies this post.

LET'S TALK VEG SNACK

Why, even though it tends to be the least appealing snack, it's important to get it in.

Raw veggies can be very hard to digest, which makes them the perfect food for signaling food in and food out. If you find you get bloated or have a hard time digesting raw veggies, then that can be a sign you are low in digestive enzymes.

Digestive enzymes build up in your digestive system by adding raw foods to your diet. They help the body process, digest and get maximum nutrients from the food you eat.

You can eat any raw veggies you like, and do not need to worry about getting in a huge variety. You can stick to the ones you like and you can mix and match.

You can also add natural dressings or dips like hummus or guacamole. You can also add cheese or nut butter.

Pickles or fermented food like cabbage also works.

You could also do a salad and use leafy greens as long as it's loaded up with raw veg. If you add raw veg to lunch you still need the afternoon snack.

If you do have a hard time digesting raw veggies, then you can cook or steam them, but do so temporarily with the goal to work your way up to eventually eating them raw.

The time between all meals and snacks should be 30 minutes to not more than 3.5 hrs. between eating.

Please take time to head over to the Facebook Group and watch the quick video that accompanies this post.

LET'S TALK NUTS AND SEEDS SNACK

Nuts and seeds can be very hard to digest, even harder than raw veggies...which is why they make the perfect afternoon snack.

Around 3-4pm the body is naturally wired to take a dip in energy. What the body is really looking for is a nap. Other places in the world refer to this as a siesta and take time to snooze.

Because most of us can't just take a nap during the day, this is where people go looking for sugar or caffeine as a pick-me-up. By adding in the nuts and or seeds, you are keeping your digestive system stimulated and working hard, which helps to keep your energy up.

The protein and fat from the nuts and seeds also helps to give you more sustaining energy, which will leave you feeling more satisfied leading up to and going into dinner. This helps keep your digestive system working hard to process and break down your larger meal, and will also help prevent you from over eating your dinner.

You can have Nuts or Seeds or a combination of both. You can use any Nuts or Seeds and ideally want to avoid oil or any salt added.

If you find them hard to digest, you can roast them or soak them.

The Nut & Seed Snack does not have an equal alternative so it is best to make a point of eating it unless you are allergic, in which case, you can *substitute with olives, beans or dairy.*

You can also add nuts and or seeds to your meals if you do, keep in mind you will still need to eat your Nut & Seed snack.

Please take time to head over to the Facebook Group and watch the quick video that accompanies this post.

LET'S TALK DINNER

Given that it's at the end of the day, try to think of dinner as more of a top-up rather than a need for fuel.

(Read that again)

**With that said, if you are not hungry for dinner, it is still best to have a small portion of it. If you are hungry for dinner, be sure to eat to satisfaction. **

Either way, make your dinner nutrient rich and use the guideline of protein being the star of the show, with veg, and leafy greens. You can also add heavier carbs IF you need, like root veg and/or grains.

Dinner can be in any combination like soup, stew, stir fry, chili, salad etc. When in doubt, go with protein and greens (cooked or raw).

Avoid using things like yogurts and oatmeal for dinner, or any kind of liquid nutrient (You can still use breakfast foods like eggs or sausage for dinner, but still incorporate the veg and greens).

There will come a time where you can have a greater variety of foods for dinner, but for now stick with the suggested components.

As with lunch, sauces, dressings, gravy, condiments, and spices can be used at will; just look for natural ingredients and avoid anything artificial.

You can also use flour in your recipes and use it for things like breading. Just do your best to avoid using excess amounts.

In terms of the timing of dinner, it is best to eat as early in your evening as possible.

Eating too late will prevent the body from following through on its wind down process, which can mess with your body's ability to get the deep and REM sleep it needs to make change.

Please take time to head over to the Facebook Group and watch the quick video that accompanies this post.

LET'S TALK FRESH EYES

Fresh eyes are key for those of you who are redoing the program to continue to reach your goal.

First, it's important to note, redoing The Program is a **VERY EFFECTIVE** method for following through and finishing the process of helping your body release fat finally and forever.

The Program works **BETTER** each time around. Not only are you more in tune, but your body is also working for you more and more.

REASONS WHY PEOPLE MIGHT STRUGGLE WITH REPEATING THE PROCESS:

1. **You have done it before, and you know you can do it again.**

   - Sometimes rather than this being an advantage or a motivator, people use it as an excuse to allow in bites of bits that you didn't allow the first time.

   - Meaning, you know how to get back on track and you know what's to come so you give yourself more wiggle room to indulge. This is an issue because you end up spending more of the process getting back on track and never gain the momentum you need to see the results you expect.

2. **You know what's coming next and expect your body to respond the same way.**

   - This is an issue because you end up disappointed that your body doesn't respond the way it did the first time around.

   - You end up assuming the process isn't working simply because it's not working the same way, the way you want, or the way you expect. Your body is different this time around and you should expect and want it to respond differently.

   - What your body connected with the first time around will be different the second, third and fourth time around. By assuming how it will respond you end up missing out on capitalizing on the areas that actually need work.

   - Meaning, you are getting in the way of your body making progress because you are trying to control what it is focusing on and how it responds.

3. **Your motivation has changed.**

   - This happens a lot when people try to use the motivation they had last time to lose weight this time.

   - Chances are what motivated you last time is not what is motivating you this time. Re-evaluating your "why" can make all the difference.

4. **You don't see an end-game.**

   - You need to see an end to the process. Leaving things open ended is not motivating and can keep you stuck in the cycle of trying to lose.

- Have a realistic time frame and plan of attack for crossing the finish line. Not only when, but also how that will feel and what it will look like.

5. **Completely missing the point that you have the advantage subsequent times around.**

- If you are repeating the process then you should be all in, stepping up your game, and using your past knowledge to challenge yourself along the way and push yourself to the max.

- You have no excuse, so perhaps that's what is holding you back, fear of being successful or fear of not following through.

- Rather than being excited about what you can do this time around, you focus on what your body isn't doing in comparison to what it was doing last time. This robs you of the opportunity to capitalize in the moment and do the best you can day to day.

Regardless of your issue, re-doing the program is an ABSOLUTE advantage, so if you are struggling, chances are it's because you are getting in your own way.

So, take a step back and assess what you need to do to step up your game. Be all in and follow through and finish!

Please take time to head over to the Facebook Group and watch the quick video that accompanies this post.

LET'S TALK SICKNESS

How to manage the plan while sick and still stay on track.

Being sick is never fun and it can be very discouraging when you are trying your best to follow the plan. Sickness always brings on detox so it can be used to your advantage so no need to worry about it setting you back.

WHAT TO DO WHEN YOU ARE SICK

1. **Drink extra water, especially if craving sugar and carbs.**

   - Resist the urge to go for crackers, white rice, bread products or sugar to settle your stomach. Sugar feeds a virus so sugar and carbs that break down into sugar are the last thing your body is looking for. Chances are what it really needs is an epic amount of water.

   - Water is essential for your body to detox out the virus, so drink as much as you can (within reason) and utilize teas and soup to get in even more liquid.

2. **Don't force the food.**

   - Chances are you won't be hungry when you are sick and that's for a reason.

   - The body is not interested in processing and digesting food, it would much rather stay focused on getting the virus out. This is a natural process that allows the body to divert all its resources into healing you.

   - The body stores a certain amount of fat for emergency purposes to use when you are sick. Your body using fat reserves for energy when you are sick is NOT the same as when you ignore hunger signals and purposely don't eat to force your body to burn fat.

   - Keep the food light and go for food that is easily digested, like soup. Be in the moment with your food choices and don't be afraid to keep it light. Once your appetite comes back, you can jump back on plan and force the formula.

   - Don't be surprised if you find your portions are naturally smaller when you resume eating. This is just your body resetting insulin sensitivity levels so go with it. It will help you fast track the process by putting you more in tune with your body's needs.

3. **Ignore the scale.**

   - Chances are your weight will be up while sick even if not eating, this is normal and happens because your body will retain the extra water it needs to get the virus out.

   - Antibiotics and medications can also have your weight up, it's not real weight gain so also not something to worry about.

   - Once your appetite comes back, your body will be looking to go into detox and that is where you will see the scale start to move.

4. **Get lots of rest**

- You don't get points for powering through. Give your body the time it needs to recover and more importantly, to rest.

- Taking naps and going to bed early will have your body bouncing back sooner than later, whereas powering through can just end up prolonging the sickness.

5. **Don't worry**

- Getting sick can feel like a major sidetrack, but it can work to your advantage. Your first priority is to feel better.

- Your body will look to rid you of the virus and make you stronger. This leads to your body working harder and fast tracking the repair and rebuild mode, which will only work to your advantage while working to lose weight.

- Once your appetite comes back, get back on track and re-establish the routine and then you can pick up where you left off and keep moving forward.

TO RECAP:

- Drink extra water.
- Keep the food light and easy to digest, don't force the formula.
- Avoid eating later in the evening which can mess with sleep.
- Have a hot epsom salt bath to help with detox.
- Take anything you need medication wise to help.
- Get lots of rest.

Please take time to head over to the Facebook Group and watch the quick video that accompanies this post.

LET'S TALK HOW TO MANAGE THE PLAN AS A DIABETIC

The program works well for all diabetics regardless of issues because the focus is on decreasing and regulating insulin while giving the body the resources & time it needs to become as healthy as possible.

It's a safe and effective program for not only weight loss but helping your body heal and address any and all health issues.

**Although I have helped many people successfully lose weight who are diabetic and this program works well and can help with diabetes, this is not an issue I personally deal with, so I asked my former client and now Vibe Ambassador, Kim Turnbull to share her firsthand experience. Please note, this is Kim's personal story. To make sure you're making the most of yours, be sure to check in with your doctor along the way if you have any questions or concerns. **

Hi all!

Thought I would share a bit about myself.

I am type 1 diabetic been on insulin for 28 years and an insulin pump for 19 Years; in 2016 found out I have rheumatoid arthritis (RA).

I have been working with Gina Livy and I wouldn't be where I am health wise without her plan and support.

Lowering the amount of insulin your body needs is the key with weight loss. The more sugar/carbs you put into your body the more your body needs insulin. The more insulin you need the more you crave sugar and the more weight you gain.

You do need carbs/sugar just not in the amount and type I was eating.

Whether your body is making the insulin or you are giving insulin the response is the same.

Before I started the program, I was taking upwards of 38-50 units a day and metformin as my body was becoming resistant to insulin, my A1C was 8.9.

Fast forward to today I am off the metformin and take 23-28 units of insulin today and my A1C was 6.5, however I have had it as low as 5.8 and I have lost weight!

My doctors could not believe the change in my weight, sugars and insulin levels.

I still have carbs, just better ones, sweet potatoes, ryvita, fruits, vegetables, almond milk, qia cereal etc. Just better food choices!

As soon as I add in something I shouldn't, I pay for it with how I feel, my weight is up not to mention my sugar!

As for my RA, I have reduced my meds. I was on 14 pills a week now I take 3 a week. And again, if I go off with my food, I can feel it.

I was a huge Diet Coke drinker and I struggled to cut it out but as Gina says it impacts metabolism and what you crave to eat.

Lowering the amount of insulin your body needs is real and has a direct impact on weight loss.

If you do take insulin or meds for diabetes, make sure you test and adjust and talk to your doctor along the way.

I test a ton to know where I am sitting, so I can minimize any high or low blood sugars.

At times I had to manage low blood sugars and dealt with them with Dex-4 tablets or some juice as advised by my doctor. Once I knew the cause of the low sugar or saw a pattern, I would make the changes in my daily insulin levels.

If my sugars run high, I look at what I am eating and watch to make sure it wasn't a rebound from a low.

Being a diabetic sometimes it isn't always about the food impacting sugars it can be stress or illness but food choices have the biggest impact on insulin levels.

Being boring and consistent helped me adjust the insulin my body needed for the food I was taking in.

This program allowed me to lose 40lbs. I have had some ups and downs and right now I am up a bit but I know why and what I need to do to give my body what it needs to drop the weight.

It is a journey but one worth the effort and ride.

I would go weeks without my weight changing and then it would drop but even though the scale wasn't always moving I could see the changes in my body.

This is just my story and what has worked for me. Learn to love being bored it works!

— with love, Kim Turnbull

**Please note: This inspirational post is not meant to replace your doctor's advice. If ever you have concerns about managing the plan, always check in with your doctor. **

LET'S TALK FERTILITY, PREGNANCY AND NURSING

The program has many benefits if you are looking to conceive, looking to lose while pregnant, looking to lose after, or while nursing.

WHAT YOU NEED TO KNOW:

Remember, this is not a diet, it's a method for helping the body focus on getting rid of fat that no longer serves a purpose. By giving the body what it needs, helping it to focus on fat loss and creating the environment for the body to follow through. All of which is done by making the body healthier in the process.

When following the Livy Method, you are helping the body decrease the weight it is used to function at as opposed to forcing the body to burn fat off by restricting calories and much needed nutrients.

The program has many benefits if you are looking to conceive, looking to lose while pregnant, or looking to lose after or while nursing

WHEN PREGNANT:

The fat that makes you fat is not needed to grow a healthy baby, so there is no reason why you can't help the body get rid of fat that no longer serves a purpose while pregnant.

In fact, growing research suggests that losing some weight during pregnancy is not only possible, it can actually be beneficial for women who are overweight or obese.

Being overweight and pregnant can come with its own set of issues you need to be mindful of. Having excess weight can cause problems during pregnancy and can lead to:

- Premature birth
- Stillbirth
- Cesarean delivery
- Heart defects in baby
- Gestational diabetes in mother (and type 2 diabetes later in life)
- High blood pressure in mother
- Preeclampsia: severe form of high blood pressure that can also affect other organs like the kidneys
- Sleep apnea
- Blood clots (especially in your legs)
- Infections in mother

Not to seem extreme. This is just to put your mind at ease. If you are looking to lose while pregnant and feeling ways about it, know that contrary to popular belief, not only can it be beneficial to lose while pregnant, for some women it's essential.

Because the program is based on helping the body become as healthy as possible by increasing nutrient absorption and addressing the body's needs, there is nothing you really need to be concerned about.

Over the next few weeks, you will be focused on giving the body what it needs, which of course is only beneficial. However, as we move forward and start making changes to the food plan, I'm sure some of you might have concerns or wonder how you should proceed.

- Firstly, continue to check in with your doctor or health care provider
- Be sure to ask as many questions as you need day to day and along the way.
- Be in tune to your body's needs.
- Even when it comes to downsizing (Week 4), which is where you start to decrease portions, you will still be eating more than enough food (eating 6-8 times a day if using bonus snacks).
- Be sure to use bonus snacks (will be introducing bonus snacks at the end of the week) as needed.

WHEN LOOKING TO CONCEIVE:

If you are dealing with fertility issues, you will find a lot of what we do here on The Program falls in line with fertility protocols.

The Program allows for healing, repairing and rebuilding, and helps the body find internal balance.

If you have been advised to take additional supplements by your fertility expert or seeing an alternative medicine expert like a Chinese medical practitioner, just be sure to keep them in the loop with any supplements you add in on plan.

WHEN NURSING:

This program tends to be great for milk supply and after the initial changes you make with the food plan, you should find you are fairly consistent in food choices so any reaction to new foods should be minimal.

Even with downsizing (Week 4), which we will discuss when the time comes, you will still be eating more than enough food to feed both you and the baby.

All the supplements we will be introducing are safe, but for good measure, check in with your doctor as they may feel differently given your personal health history.

In fact, if you have any concerns along the way, be sure to check in with your doctor and make sure you are asking any questions you have day to day on the Questions Post.

Please take time to head over to the Facebook Group and watch the quick video that accompanies this post.

LET'S TALK CRAVINGS

At this point, if you are following The Program, you should find any cravings you had or have are minimal. And if you do have them, they are nothing to be feared.

**Cravings are just simply a message from the body. They are the body's way of communicating it's needs by associating the foods that can help get it what it wants. **

If you are following the Food Plan, drinking the water, and taking the supplements, any cravings should be few and far between. And if they do pop up, it's usually just a matter of making a few tweaks.

LET'S TALK SUGAR:

The key to beating sugar cravings is to understand that it's not actually sugar people are addicted to; it's the high insulin levels needed to break it down that has you reaching for sweets.

WHY?

- Insulin is the hormone that allows your body to use glucose for energy. Glucose is a type of sugar found in carbs like fruits, vegetables, and naturally occurring sugar that your body uses for energy. After you eat food and your digestive system breaks it down, your pancreas releases insulin to help regulate your blood sugar.

- When you reach for the sweets or foods with high sugar content, your body can flood with too much insulin, which causes your blood glucose levels to drop. This creates a dip in energy and a desire for even more sugar.

- This can create a vicious cycle that makes taking sugar and carbs out of your diet a challenge.

WHY AM I CRAVING SO MUCH SUGAR IN THE FIRST PLACE?

LET'S BREAK IT DOWN:

1. **More is more:**

- When you have sugar, your body will immediately want more sugar. These cravings can be so intense that if you create a habit of having sugar at the same time every day, your body will begin to crave and expect it at that same time daily. This is also the reason you end up eating that whole box of cookies in one sitting!

THE FIX:

- Add some protein and fat.

- Making sure to add in healthy fats to your meals along with protein, will help to prevent any cravings along the way.

- But if you do find yourself indulging, you can neutralize sugar cravings by having some protein and fat with your sweet treat. For example, if you indulge in a cookie, you can cut the desire to eat another cookie by having a slice of cheese or a handful of nuts.

- The protein and fat will help neutralize the amount of insulin your body uses to break down the sugar and decrease your cravings, giving your will power a fighting chance to kick in and help.

2. **Dehydration is a factor:**

- When you are dehydrated and not picking up on the cues from your body to drink more, your body's next best bet is to crave foods with a high-water content, like fruit. Fruits are also sweet, so you may mistake your body's cue to consume more water and instead find yourself reaching for processed carbs and sugar.

- This is why you may hear the advice to drink a glass of water before you eat to satisfy your appetite. It doesn't satisfy your appetite, but if it's water that you actually need, you may realize you are not really hungry after all.

THE FIX:

- Drink more water.

- Sip water throughout the day, aiming for a minimum of 3.5 litres a day and even more on days you exercise or are more active.

3. **You are tired:**

- When you are tired, your body goes looking for a pick-me-up, and you may find yourself reaching for something sweet.

- The same thing happens around 3 or 4 p.m. each afternoon when the body is wired to take a drop in energy and slows your circadian rhythm. What your body is really looking for is a nap. (There are places in the world that do just that: think of the siesta.)

- In our fast-paced, high-stress world, it's not always possible to take a nice afternoon nap, so the body goes looking for easy energy by way of higher sugar to pick it up and keep it going.

THE FIX:

- Make sure to eat all your meals and especially your snacks. This will help to avoid energy levels that dip when you go for long periods of time without eating.

- Your mid-morning snack of fresh fruit will top up your energy reserves in the morning and your raw veggies, nuts and seeds in the afternoon will keep your body working hard throughout the afternoon.

- These foods have a high nutrient value and are harder to digest, which will keep your digestion stimulated and your body awake and functioning when it's craving a nap.

- With a few adjustments, you can easily beat the need for sweets and stay on track to reach your goals and not be held captive by sugar cravings anymore!

LET'S TALK SALT:

When you crave sugar, it generally means that you need more water. When you crave salt, it generally means that the body is asking for more good fat. When you are stressed, your body is revving high, you burn lots of calories, your brain works really hard and your body quickly gets depleted of its nutrients.

Periods of high stress can rapidly deplete your vitamin and mineral reserves. So, when you are stressed, your body is looking for more sustaining energy by way of good fat.

You don't have to be stressed for the body to need more good fat. Fat is essential for cellular function as well as brain and heart health. It also works like a transport system for your body to process and digest carbs and protein.

Your body would rather get that fat from the foods you eat than to utilize its emergency reserve. Without enough good fat coming in, your body will be reluctant to let go of the fat that makes you fat. So, one way you can speed up that fat loss process is to make sure you are getting lots of good fats in your meals and adding in an omega 3.

LET'S TALK TUMMY RUMBLINGS & HUNGER PAINS:

We are taught to believe if your tummy rumbles you must be hungry, when in fact that's not what the noise and rumblings are about. It's actually your body's natural MMC or Migrating Motor Complex.

Your digestive system works like a self-cleaning oven where, in between processing and digesting food, it works to clear bacteria and food particles out of the small intestine.

Because we are eating so often during the day, the body is doing most of this work at night. As we move through the program, we will be phasing you into more natural patterns of eating which will be more in tune to your body's needs, which include the downtime it needs in between meals to self-regulate.

TO RECAP:

Cravings are nothing to stress about, though they can give you great insight into your body's needs. Usually, the smallest tweak or adjustments can make all the difference.

It's important to note it's not about controlling your cravings; it's about being in tune to them. As you progress through the program, you will become more in tune and able to differentiate between the body's needs and your wants.

You may also find yourself craving other kinds of foods and even specific foods. At the end of this process, your body will clearly let you know when it's hungry, what it's hungry for, and how much you need to eat.

Paying attention to those cravings can help you better meet your body's needs so that your body can focus on what you need…and get the fat out.

Please take time to head over to the Facebook Group and watch the quick video that accompanies this post.

NUTRIENT RICH MEALS

By now I'm sure you have heard us say "Make your meals nutrient rich". But do you know what that really means? I'm going to use a salad as an example, but the same idea can be applied to absolutely ANY meal.

LET'S BREAK IT DOWN...

- Spring Mix/Greens = leafy greens + roughage + vitamins + minerals + protein
- Variety of Vegetables = fiber + vitamins
- Avocado = healthy fat + potassium + fiber
- Feta cheese = healthy fat + protein
- Nuts and Seeds = healthy fat + protein
- Honey Mustard Vinaigrette = healthy fat because it's made with olive oil (plus it's delicious!)

Are you picking up what I'm laying down? A simple, small salad loaded up with stuff, not only provides you with a variety of nutrients, but is also more sustaining!

**Look for quality over quantity and you will soon find that you don't need as much food to feel satisfied. **

Nutrient rich meals provide the most bang for your buck and give you longer lasting energy.

Even if you can just sneak in one or two extra things like a drizzle of olive oil, an extra veg, or a few nuts... it can make all the difference.

THINGS TO HAVE ON HAND THAT CAN QUICKLY BUMP UP YOUR MEALS:

These are some items that I always have on hand to quickly and easily level up my meals when something is lacking.

- A variety of nuts and seeds - good fat and protein are an excellent addition to yogurt or oats
- Olives - good fat
- Pickled and marinated veg like artichoke hearts, pickled beets, roasted red peppers, etc. - bump up your veggies.
- Good quality oils like extra virgin olive oil, nut oils, avocado and coconut oil - good fats
- Quality salad dressings (store bought or homemade)
- Coconut milk - a great healthy fat addition to things like your morning oatmeal or cereal.
- Salsa - extra veg
- Guacamole - good fat

- Hummus - good fat plus protein
- Tuna, sardines, smoked oysters - I always have these in the cupboard as a quick way to add protein to any meal.

Now go forth and eat RICH!

Please take time to head over to the Facebook Group and watch the quick video that accompanies this post.

LET'S TALK WEIGHT LOSS

And get real about it.

Before talking about numbers on the scale, please make time to read the post about **THE SCALE**. There, I talk about the fact that the scale is going to **FLUCTUATE**.

I talk about what real weight loss looks like, the fact the scale goes up before it goes down, and that is not only NORMAL in most cases, it's to be expected.

I also give a lot of reasons why the scale would be up, like water retention & dehydration, salty or hard to digest food, detox & hormone balancing… to name a few. None of which have anything to do with real weight gain. And most of which are a sign your body is about to start dropping fat.

The sooner you understand that the body is not trying to make you fat, the less stressed you are going to be throughout this process.

IT IS IMPORTANT TO UNDERSTAND:

- It is impossible to make fat overnight.
- It is impossible for the body to make fat over the weekend.
- And you would be hard-pressed to make fat over a week.
- Your body converting the food you eat into fat that makes you fat is a complicated and complex process and takes longer than you think.
- You have signed up for a weight loss program. A very effective one. You are going to lose weight.

THIS IS NOT ABOUT A QUICK FIX:

- We're into healthy, maintainable weight loss.
- Most of you are here because you know someone who has been successful in losing weight with the Program. You will be just as successful if you show up every day and do the work for as long as it takes to get the job done. Remember that might look different than the person who inspired you to join.
- We are not focused on numbers on the scale in the first few weeks. And you will find I'm not keen to even talk about it until we start to focus on it.
- If the scale moves in the first few weeks, great! And if it doesn't, I'm not worried. As frustrating as that is going to be for some of you, it's true.

Make no mistake, I am here to help you lose a lot of weight and make life changing changes, but that takes time and there is a process to it. Losing weight can be unnerving at times and can have you feeling overwhelmed and even hopeless, especially if you have a lot of weight to lose. The feelings and emotions you have about weight loss are very real and I want you to know that I take that seriously.

I want to make sure you are all clear and feeling confident about this process so please take time to head over to the Facebook Group and watch the quick video where I talk about expectations, what weight loss will look like, and things you need to keep in mind when it comes to the numbers on the scale.

Please take time to head over to the Facebook Group and watch the quick video that accompanies this post.

WONDERING WHY YOUR WEIGHT IS UP?

While following the Plan, your weight might go up for various reasons, none of which will have anything to do with actual weight gain.

**Let me be clear...if following the Plan, eating all the meals and snacks, making foods nutrient rich and eating to satisfaction (or even overeating) you are NOT going to gain weight. **

The body is not inclined to want to store fat, in fact it's quite the opposite. The body wants your fat gone as much as you do! It's important to understand that throughout this Program, your weight is going to naturally fluctuate, no matter what you do.

REASONS YOUR WEIGHT CAN BE UP:

- Stress
- Lack of sleep
- Salty food
- Hard to digest food (like red meat, although not a reason to not eat it)
- Dehydration
- Body fighting an illness
- Body sore from a workout
- Body reacting to change in routine
- Body reacting to change in food
- Body reacting to new medication or change in medications
- Body reacting to any new supplements or change in supplements
- Deficiencies like being low in iron
- Hormones balancing
- PMS
- Your scale needing new batteries
- And the last, and most important reason, is your body is detoxing and your weight is about to drop.

**If you haven't seen it yet, take time to review the scale post and watch the video (posted in the Facebook Support Group) as it's important to understand what real weight loss looks like on the scale. **

If you stick around and keep showing up, you are going to be successful and lose your weight regardless of the little ups along the way. The ups are normal and to be expected. Although we do like to have fun around here, weight loss can have its frustrating moments so we don't want anyone stressing about the scale any more than they need to...or even at all!

Hope this helps. Embrace the little ups because they always lead to the big drops!

Please take time to head over to the Facebook Group and watch the quick video that accompanies this post.

LET'S TALK WHAT TO DO IF YOU ARE NOT HUNGRY

With all the changes the body is making in the first few weeks, it's normal to feel hungrier.

However, it's also normal to not feel hungry.

Over the last few weeks, you have been working hard to give your body everything it needs so that it no longer feels the need to store fat. By being consistent and following the food plan, you are addressing your cravings and naturally helping the body reduce portion sizes without even trying.

This will lead to a change in your appetite as the body will be working hard to regulate your metabolism & blood sugar, as well as making internal and external changes and balancing hormones.

As your body works hard to make change and works hard to find balance, these changes will have your hunger levels changing day to day and week to week. Which is why it is normal to not feel hungry for meals and snacks. One day you might be hungry every 5 mins and then the next day, 5 hours can go by and you won't be hungry at all.

WHICH BRINGS US TO THE QUESTION...WHY DO YOU HAVE TO EAT WHEN YOU ARE NOT HUNGRY?

- During the day, the routine is key. We are still in the early stages of making the body feel confident it is going to get what it needs so it doesn't feel the need to store fat. Therefore, you need to eat! Even if just a small token amount.

- Consistency helps to maintain and reinforce the routine of the Food Plan Formula. This will play a key role moving forward and with managing your weight loss.

- There are many benefits to eating a token amount of your meals and snacks even if you are not hungry. Having a small token amount of food signals food in and food out, which aids indigestion and helps with processing food in and out.

- Eating makes your body work hard to process and digest food which helps to boost metabolism and improves digestion.

- Being consistent helps to manage your hunger levels...since food takes time to digest you are being proactive in managing your appetite.

WHEN IT COMES TO DINNER:

- There will come a time when you can skip dinner, but for now it's best you have something small.

- Stick with some leafy greens and protein if not hungry and just eat a token amount.

- Along with reinforcing the routine, it also helps to prevent the urge to snack later.

As we progress, we will be making changes to the Food Plan that will continually shake things up and in turn, have your appetite all over the place.

Next week, for example, we will be focused on being as consistent as possible. Consistent to the point of boredom which will help you work through any issues of utilizing food for anything other than nutritional needs.

You are going to notice that some days you will be hungrier than others, which is totally normal and why the focus right now is to eat all meals and snacks, make your food choices nutrient rich, and eat to satisfaction regardless of what that portion looks like.

Bottom line: if you are not hungry, then still eat a small token amount.

**Token amounts means just enough food to stimulate your digestive system so at least 4-5 bites of food with 4-5 chews each bite, give or take. **

Please take time to head over to the Facebook Group and watch the quick video that accompanies this post.

LET'S TALK ABOUT HUNGER

What it means to be hungry and the difference between true hunger vs. your body craving certain foods, your energy draining, hormones balancing, and detox.

As we work this week to fine tune and perfect the Plan, some of you will be introducing bonus snacks as a way to manage hunger levels. I'm hoping this breakdown will give you more clarity as to if and when you need to add in the bonus snacks and when you can hold off till it's time to eat your regularly scheduled meals and snacks.

THE MOST IMPORTANT THING YOU NEED TO UNDERSTAND ABOUT HUNGER:

- Hunger is the way your body checks in with you and lets you know where it's at and what it needs throughout the day.

- Hunger is just another way the body communicates its needs, a "heads up" kind of thing, more than an immediate need for food.

- The body knows that food can take hours to process and digest through your system. Therefore, it takes that into account when giving you a heads up on when you need to eat.

- Periodically throughout the day and into the evening your body will do a "systems check" and will let you know when it's time to start thinking about eating based on its current energy reserve.

If you are dealing with hunger in-between meals & snacks, or in the evening, be sure to refer to the video that accompanies this post. As we move forward in the program, we will continue to talk a lot more about hunger, the timing, portions and nutrients needed to properly address your body's changing hunger levels.

Please take time to head over to the Facebook Group and watch the quick video that accompanies this post.

HOW TO ADVOCATE FOR YOURSELF

As our first official week begins, we want to help set you up for the best success moving forward. We have thrown a lot of information at you over the past few days and we understand that it's a lot to take in.

But remember... if you want to be successful you must read over the posts and watch the videos, to understand all the info. The videos expand on the written post so don't miss the extra tidbits provided within them. The information we provide in this Program is EVERYTHING. You must educate yourself so you can have a deeper understanding of how your body works. Then use it to GET THE FAT OUT!

Many other diets and weight loss programs out there are designed to spoon-feed and handhold. Telling you exactly what to eat, how much, on which days, and which meals etc. It has trained many of us to feel lost in thinking for ourselves when it comes to food, eating, and our bodies in general. We have become out of touch because of so much misinformation and old, archaic dieting bull-crap!

This Program takes you through a process that puts you back in tune with your body and teaches you how to think for yourself and listen to your body's cues...and that takes effort.

It is your "job" to read all the information and understand it as much as possible. Think of it as studying for an exam.

It might not make much sense right now but trust me, it all comes together in the end. It's a process and this Program is about so much more than weight loss. It's an epic course in getting to know YOU!

WHICH BRINGS ME TO THE QUESTIONS.

Although we are happy to answer all the questions you have, we are expecting those questions to be based on the information you have already read and listened to.

Given that this is the first week, and it's a lot of information, we understand that not everyone has had time to read everything over and watch the accompanying videos. Check into the Facebook Group and USE THOSE GUIDES to keep track of what you have read and/or watched.

Go back to Day 1 and work your way up to today. BE SURE YOU READ OVER EVERYTHING and watch the video content (found in the Facebook Group). We understand that many of you have very busy schedules and it can take some time to get to the info. So, of course, we are more than happy to answer your questions, but also keep in mind, if you want to be successful and lose weight, you need to also make the time. You do not have to watch the Facebook Lives but if you can watch at least some of them, I can assure you, it will be very beneficial. Gina always goes into great detail to answer some of the questions asked during the Lives. Put your earbuds on and listen while you're cooking or cleaning the house, taking a walk...or relaxing in the bath!

Your job is to:

- Review the info in the Welcome, Food Plan and Prep Week Guides.

- Read all the posts and watch the informational videos.

- Take notes.

- Ask your questions AFTER reviewing the information.

- If you think of a new question, ask yourself if this has already been covered and go look for that post or posts, and read them over before asking your question. 9 times out of 10 the answer is there but it's been overlooked. Finding the answer yourself helps to better retain it.

You can't make epic changes without doing the work! We take weight loss seriously and we expect you will too! Make the time for yourself. You owe it to yourself. You deserve to be successful and feel amazing!

Now go start studying for this epic, life changing course so you can nail it!

5 PRO TIPS TO BE MORE PROACTIVE WITH THIS PROCESS

As we move forward, you are going to hear me talk a lot about being proactive with this process. So, I thought I would break it down and put together some tips for making the most of my Program from this point.

Proactive adjective

pro·ac·tive (proh-ak-tiv)

"Definition of proactive 1 [proentry 2 + reactive]: acting in anticipation of future problems, needs, or changes"

1. **Make sure you are watching the videos that go along with the posts**

   - The written information is only a short summary. In the videos, I go more in-depth and might also touch on other elements not listed.

   - The more you understand the process, the more you will see it all coming together. When you can understand the process, it makes it so much easier to follow… which makes it so much more effective in the end.

2. **Be sure to keep up with the GUIDES**

   - Guides are where all of the information is posted day to day. Not all of the information is included in the Workbook such as any videos, live content, share pages etc. You can click "Done" at the end of each post to easily keep track of what you have reviewed and anything new.

3. **Use TOPICS button and the SEARCH**

   - You can use the Topics button or search using the magnifying glass at the top of the Group Page to quickly search & review any post or topic from past guides. Make sure you are searching in the group, not Facebook in general.

   - Between all the Posts and all the questions and answers, the search bar can be quite handy.

   - Using the Search bar literally searches every word posted in the group …so if you search water, any post or conversation about water will pop up.

4. **From this point the program moves fast, so show up every day**

   - Each week, the focus will change and you will be making changes to the Food Plan. The changes you make week to week become the jumping off point for the following week.

- Because there is no going back (and you don't want to keep looking back), the goal is to be all in and keep things moving forward.
- Set your intention in the morning and check in with yourself at the end of the day, taking note of where you excelled and any areas that could use more attention.

5. **Continue to ask questions**

- Some weeks can be tricky, and some days are sure to be better than others. Because it can be easy to get sidetracked with this process for so many reasons, if you are ever unsure at any point on how to proceed, let us know.
- Don't spend time guessing or hoping you are doing the right thing. It's key to be clear on what you need to do each week so don't be shy about asking questions.

A BONUS TIP: Keep a journal and use our new app for tracking how your body is responding to the process. Journals (see Journaling Post) can help with any problem solving should it be needed along the way and give you great insight into how to make the most out of this process.

LET'S TALK KEEPING A JOURNAL/USING OUR NEW APP

Why it can be a great idea to be tracking your progress along the way.

BENEFITS OF JOURNALING

A journal can be a great tool to help give you insight into how your body is responding to the process.

It can help you pick up on patterns of behavior and responses, and give you a better idea of what weight loss looks like specifically to you.

It can help you pick up on any food sensitivities, especially if you have digestive issues. It can help you track bowel movements if you struggle in that department.

It can help you track your body's response to the supplements, or anything new you are adding in or taking out.

It can also help to track your mood and can be beneficial in helping you show up for yourself every day, by taking time to think about how you are managing your emotions and how you are feeling day to day.

THINGS TO TRACK

- Weight in the morning
- How you are feeling physically and mentally
- Food
- Water
- Extras (added food and drink on or not on plan)
- Bowel movements if they are an issue
- Notable responses from food
- Digestive upset
- Sleep
- Medications
- Supplements
- Notable wins not food related
- Energy day to day
- Changes taking place that aren't scale related

You can use good old pen and paper, your computer, or our new app. Whatever works best for you!

Not so much now, but as we progress, your journal can be a very helpful tool to problem solve in conjunction with the info being posted in the group.

The more tools the better!

Please take time to head over to the Facebook Group and watch the quick video that accompanies this post.

LET'S TALK ABOUT BONUS SNACKS

If you need them and when to add them in.

As we wind down this first official week of The Program, it's time to look ahead to Week 2, which will have you fine tuning and perfecting The Plan.

During the first week, you ate in a way that allows your body to adjust to lower insulin levels, which, in turn, will help to decrease the amount of food you will need to feel satisfied.

For Week 2, you are going to continue to follow the Food Plan but the focus will be on making adjustments day to day, so you feel more satisfied at the end of each day.

THIS IS WHERE BONUS SNACKS COME IN.

**Bonus snacks are extra snacks that can be used by those of you who are up super early, those of you who are more physical in your day (super active job), or for those long shift turnarounds where you are awake for 24hrs. **

First, it's key to note that Bonus Snacks are NOT meant to replace your regular snacks, so you will still need to eat them. And you cannot switch out your regularly scheduled snacks for bonus snacks.

Please note: If you are continually skipping breakfast and having to add in bonus snacks then you should be eating breakfast.

Bonus snacks are to be added **ONLY if needed** for nutritional requirements because you are feeling hungry...they do not need to be added in every day.

THE TIMING OF THE BONUS SNACKS IS VERY SPECIFIC:

1.   Can be added in between your morning fruit snack and lunch.

2.   Can be added between your lunch and raw veg snack. For example:

- Protein for breakfast
- Fruit for morning snack
- BONUS SNACK
- Lunch
- BONUS SNACK
- Raw veg
- Nuts/seeds
- Dinner

The timing between these snacks and the rest is the same; 30 minutes to 3.5 hours.

WHAT YOU CAN HAVE FOR BONUS SNACKS:

MORNING BONUS SNACK:

- Yogurt or other dairy products, such as cottage cheese or other cheeses
- More fruit with nuts, seeds, nut butter, cheese or any protein and fat
- Vegetables raw or cooked and you can add dip or cheese
- Boiled egg or any other protein
- Half of your lunch eaten early
- Ryvita/high fiber cracker with spread (only if not used at breakfast)
- Shake with protein, veg or fruit and added fat (be mindful of portion size)

AFTERNOON BONUS SNACK:

- Can be any of the above except nuts & seeds.

Keep in mind, if you add in the bonus snacks and find yourself not hungry for your regular snacks, you still need to eat them even if you keep the portion small.

I recognize it may seem counterintuitive to eat more when trying to lose weight, but right now it is key to address why your body is feeling a need to store fat and to be more in tune with its needs.

This is the quickest and most effective way to get the body to focus on fat loss.

Some of you, depending on how early you get up or how active you are, may need to utilize the bonus snacks more often while others may not.

Please take time to head over to the Facebook Group and watch the quick video that accompanies this post.

LET'S TALK WEEKENDS

Why they are nothing to worry about and how to make the most of them.

When it comes to weight loss, it can seem like there is always something getting in the way and throwing you off track; birthdays, holidays, vacation days, let alone just your average weekend.

Lack of routine, travel, eating off foods like salty food, hard to digest food, high sugar content foods, lack of water, and even lack of sleep can easily have your weight up.

Good thing it's not as easy as you think to gain weight, and it takes a lot longer than you think for your body to convert the food you eat into actual fat. So, when you find the scale creeping up after a little indulging, chances are it's not real weight gain.

Which is why I always say there is nothing you can do in a weekend or even a few weeks that can't be undone by getting back at it!

Having off weekends and going off Plan is going to happen, for the sake of weight loss, you want to keep those days to a minimum. But with that said, there is also nothing to stress about.

Staying as consistent as possible is key, but if you get off track just get right back on track, because as long as you stay in the game and keep showing up, you are going to get there.

Please take time to head over to the Facebook Group and watch the quick video that accompanies this post.

LET'S TALK GOAL WEIGHT

People always ask me what's a good goal weight?

Without sounding cliché, I really do think it's when you feel comfortable in your own skin.

With that said though, a good baseline I use for clients is your lowest weight after the age of 21 that you were able to easily maintain.

That doesn't mean if you have always carried extra weight that you can't weigh less than you ever have... because you totally can. A lot of people have had weight issues from childhood but that doesn't mean you can't be successful at losing or losing a lot.

Once you address why your body is feeling the need to store fat (like we are doing in the first few weeks), the body will be happy to get rid of it, regardless of when you gained or how long you have carried the extra weight.

People think genetics plays a role, but it doesn't. People who have genetically more fat cells may have the capacity to gain more when they do gain, but that doesn't mean it's harder for them to lose.

I know that it's easier said than done but focusing on all the positive changes that come with weight loss can be more motivating than aiming for a certain number on the scale.

Also, when it comes to that number on the scale, I suggest you ditch the BMI charts and the old archaic means of measuring what your weight should be. There are so many variables that they don't account for. Instead, go by how you feel and aim to be as healthy as possible regardless of weight.

It can be good to set a target weight as a goal, but it can also just add more stress. Visualizing looking and feeling your best can be just as, if not more, effective.

When it comes down to numbers, I find most people underestimate out of fear of failing. Because with this Program, weight loss is such a process, it is normal to find yourself setting new goals along the way.

Please take time to head over to the Facebook Group and watch the quick video that accompanies this post.

WEEK 1 RECAP AND A SNEAK PEEK INTO WEEK 2

As the first official week of the program comes to an end, I want to touch base and check in to see how you are doing!

LET'S TALK ABOUT MOTIVATION AND SUCCESS.

I recognize that for many of you the journey to lose weight thus far has been a frustrating one, having spent a lot of time, energy and money on diets. Because of that, please know that I am always super mindful about this program not being one more thing you have tried that didn't work.

I also understand that some of the things I am suggesting seem far removed from traditional diets, which I view as a good thing, since traditional diets don't work.

If you stick around, what you are learning and how your body is responding will start to come together and, not only will it make a lot of sense, but it will also help you lose a lot of weight.

Even if you feel like you have already messed up, are behind, or you are feeling apprehensive about moving forward, this program takes all those things into account.

Although I like to set the bar high, there is no such thing as "perfect" with this program because weight loss is a process. I always say, "there is never a good time to lose weight". There is always going to be something getting in the way, like holidays, birthdays, and times in life when the desire to lose weight may seem trivial in comparison to what you have going on.

Even though life keeps getting in the way, the desire to lose weight doesn't go away because I believe for most of you, this Process is not just about vanity and fitting into a pair of jeans. It's about being in tune with your body's needs and feeling comfortable in your skin as well as being as healthy and happy as you can possibly be.

As you move forward week to week, continue to check in each day, watch the check in video and review all of the information. I am a big believer in having a deeper level of understanding, so if you have questions or need clarification, please never hesitate to ask!

My only concern, moving forward, is that you stay in the game, and you keep showing up, even on the days you want to give up. There absolutely WILL BE moments of frustration, but for the most part, we truly believe this process can be fun!

LOSING WEIGHT IS NOT A PUNISHMENT. IT'S A JOURNEY IN SELF LOVE AND LIVING YOUR BEST LIFE!

I have seen great things happen and amazing life changes take place when people put time and energy into giving their bodies what it needs to make lasting changes.

Chances are, you are here because somewhere along the way your body got the message it needed to store fat and that message has been reinforced time and time again over the years. This is why the first few weeks of The Program are all about giving the body what it needs.

Although many of you have already been experiencing fat loss, know that if you haven't, it's nothing to be concerned about. It might be frustrating, but it's also perfectly normal.

We have a long way to go, and everyone's body will respond differently. It isn't until Week 3/4 that we even start to focus on fat loss. If you have faith in The Process, take it day by day, and do the work, then you will be successful regardless of how quickly you start to lose.

A SNEAK PEEK AT WEEK 2

Week 2 is more of the same but with the focus on fine tuning and perfecting...as your body adjusts to the changes that you have already made.

In Week 2, you will continue to focus on giving your body what it needs so it no longer feels the need to store fat. The focus is all about making adjustments, so you are feeling satisfied at the end of the day.

In the first few weeks, by following the basic Food Plan, you are eating in a way that will allow your body to adjust to lower insulin levels, which will eventually lead to you naturally feeling more satisfied on smaller portions.

With that said though, you are not to try to eat less. Be open to your body's needs day to day and continue to eat to satisfaction. For example, one day you might need one egg to feel satisfied and then the next day you might need three.

The goal is to eat to satisfaction, not to TRY to eat less.

In fact, as you enter into Week 2, you may find your appetite has increased because of your increasing metabolism. So in order to satisfy this increased hunger, we have introduced Bonus Snacks. Be sure to read over the Bonus Snacks post, watch the video, and ask any questions you have.

At the beginning of Week 2, I will be introducing Supplements.

These can play a key role in this process and help the body drop fat. Supplements can help where the body is deficient, which can make all the difference when it comes to addressing the body's needs and speeding up the weight loss process.

WEEK 2 GUIDELINES: FINE TUNING AND PERFECTING

Week 2 has you fine tuning and perfecting the changes you made in Week 1. As well as adding in Bonus Snacks and implementing the suggested supplements if needed.

Last week was all about implementing the changes you needed to make with the Food Plan and letting the body adjust.

This week is all about Fine Tuning & Perfecting the changes you have made so far.

THE GOAL FOR THIS WEEK:

- Eat all meals and snacks
- Make all food choices as nutrient rich as possible
- Eat to satisfaction
- Add in BONUS snacks IF needed
- Be as consistent as possible

The idea behind fine tuning and perfecting is making sure you feel satisfied at the end of the day.

So, if you are feeling full and stuffed at the end of the day, you want to pay extra attention to the portions the next day. And alternatively, if you are hungry at the end of the day, be sure to eat your meals and snacks (don't skip breakfast), make your foods as nutrient rich as possible, and use Bonus Snacks if needed.

Bonus snacks are extra snacks that you can add in if you find you are continuously feeling unsatisfied at the end of the day, or your appetite is increasing because your metabolism is increasing.

Bonus snacks are to be added ONLY if needed for nutritional requirements because you are feeling hungry not because you "feel like" a snack.

**As a reminder, Bonus Snacks are NOT meant to replace your regular snacks so you will still need to keep those in. **

Keep in mind, you can keep your food choices simple, or you can make them as fancy as you like if cooking is something you enjoy.

Even when keeping things simple, don't be afraid to add in and bump your meals with a variety of nutrient rich ingredients.

It's not always about adding in more food, sometimes it's about eating the right food.

Along with Veggies, cheese, dips, sauces and any of your favorite condiments or spices can be added as long as they are made with good quality ingredients. You can load up salads and make your soups, stews, and stir-fry with tons of fresh foods and flavours and if you prefer plain, then that's ok too!

Week 2 also has us introducing SUPPLEMENTS that can play a key role in this process.

Supplements can help where the body is deficient, which can make all the difference when it comes to addressing the body's needs and speeding up the weight loss process.

While working on fine tuning and perfecting the Food Plan, water intake & supplements this week, we will also be covering a variety of topics in the Group.

Be sure to check into the Facebook Group every day, utilize the GUIDES to see what is being posted day to day and, as always, if you have questions be sure to let us know.

Please take time to head over to the Facebook Group and watch the quick video that accompanies this post.

LET'S TALK SUPPLEMENTS

The following are basic supplements that, over the years, I have found helpful to aid in deficiencies in the body that may affect your ability to drop weight and/or can help speed up the process. These supplements are suggested because in my experience they can help and work well with The Program and weight loss.

**It's up to you to decide if you want to add them in. We aren't trying to push supplements on anyone and understand that some may not be able to take them or afford all of them. **

We do not work with any supplement companies and do not make money from selling or promoting them. I will not ask you to buy any supplements from any specific company and if I do suggest a specific brand, it is because it is my personal preference or simply a good example. There are a ton of great brands at a variety of price points.

**Please note that if you have any concerns with these supplements interacting with the current medications you are taking or for any other reason, consult your family doctor. **

Before we get started:

- I'm not partial to any particular brands and even suggest switching up brands every now and then to find one that works best for you. I will often switch mine up based on what is on sale.

- I suggest getting to know the people at your local health food store and/or pharmacy to help make the best choice for you.

- Take time to read over all of the information a few times and be sure to ask any questions you need to be clear on what to look for, or things to keep in mind when purchasing any products.

- The supplements I am about to suggest are, in my experience, beneficial to weight loss because when you are deficient in them, it can affect your ability to lose weight and achieve maximum results in the time frame we are working with.

- Although they are all beneficial to the human body and basic health in general, before you run out and buy them for the sake of weight loss, I want you to understand why they are a benefit and assess if they are right for you.

**If you are unsure about any interaction with health issues you have or medication you take, be sure to check with your doctor. **

BASIC SUPPLEMENT LIST

PROBIOTICS

A probiotic is good bacteria added to your digestive system that helps promote a healthy immune system, but more importantly for our purpose, helps with weight loss by improving digestion.

Digestion is important for weight loss because if your body is unable to process food properly and get the nutrients your body needs, it will store fat to compensate or be reluctant to let it go.

- Probiotics come in pill, powdered, or liquid form.

- The probiotic added to foods like yogurt is usually not sufficient enough.

- I suggest looking for a "one a day" with higher potency. This helps minimize the number of pills you have to take each day. Probiotics come in a variety of different potencies and strains and also price ranges.

Look for a probiotic with a variety of strains, especially:

- L. acidophilus

- B. Longum

- B. bifidum

- L. rhamnose

- L. fermentum

If you feel you have digestive issues, issues with bowel movements or suffer from chronic health issues and/or skin issues, we suggest investing in a higher quality probiotic, usually found in the refrigerated section. If you don't feel you have these issues, then you are just looking for one to cover the bases.

DOSE

5-10 billion CFUs is an average potency. Follow the recommended dosage on your product's label.

WHEN TO TAKE

Take either on an empty stomach 30 mins before breakfast or with breakfast. The advantage of taking with or without food is debatable. You can also take it before bed. Whichever time you choose, try to be consistent with it. Avoid taking after a meal.

PLEASE NOTE: If you're following SIBO or the FODMAP diet while also following the plan, you might be advised NOT to add in a probiotic. If unsure, always check in with your healthcare provider.

PROBIOTIC FOOD SOURCES

- Yogurt

- Kefir

- Buttermilk

- Some cheeses such as Gouda, Cheddar, Parmesan and Swiss

- Sauerkraut

- Kimchi

- Pickles that are naturally fermented like Strubbs. If they contain vinegar they aren't naturally fermented.
- Tempeh
- Miso
- Kombucha be mindful of sugar content

VITAMIN D, D3:

Vitamin D is beneficial for weight loss because it tricks the body into thinking it is summer year-round, eliminating the need for the body to hold on to the extra fat it feels inclined to store over the winter months. It is also essential in supporting the body's metabolism.

Low levels of vitamin D are often found in people who have weight to lose because when someone is lacking Vit D, the hypothalamus (the very small part of your brain that regulates hormonal functions, amongst other things) senses low vitamin D levels and responds by increasing body weight.

- Vit D comes in drops or pills. I like drops but pills work.
- Vit D2 is the vegan form
- Vit D3 is the most effective for raising levels as it absorbs better.
- It is better absorbed if taken with a meal that contains fat.

DOSE

600-2000 IU/day is the recommended dose range. Follow package directions for dose.

WHEN TO TAKE

Take with breakfast or lunch because taking it too late in the day can interrupt the body's production of melatonin and mess with your sleep.

ALTERNATE SOURCES FOR VITAMIN D:

Very few foods contain any significant amounts of vitamin D so sun exposure is our best source if not supplementing.

According to the Vitamin D Council, a person with light skin needs approximately 15 minutes of sun exposure and a dark skin person needs a couple of hours.

- Your skin produces more vitamin D from the sun during mid-day, when the sun is at its highest point.
- The more skin that is exposed the more vitamin D the body will make.
- Darker skin takes longer to make vitamin D than paler skin.

OMEGA 3:

If your body is feeling a need to store fat, one way you can speed up the fat loss process is to add in more good fat. Without enough good fat coming in, the body will be reluctant to let go of the stored fat that it keeps around for emergency purposes.

30% of your diet should come from fat and ideally 10% of that should come from omega 3. The primary source of omega 3 is fish and unless you are eating a lot of it, it can be difficult for the body to get enough.

Best taken with food and ideally higher fat for best absorption. Because it can be hard to digest, you can divide the dose and take it at breakfast or lunch. Some find refrigerating or even freezing the capsules makes it easier to digest. Follow package directions for dose.

- Omega 3 comes in pill or liquid (oil). Both are equally good.
- If you don't like fish oil you can use vegan alternatives like a 3-6-9 combo.
- I would also look for a high potency one-a-day, again, to minimize the number of pills to take in a day.

DOSE

500-3000 mg per day is the recommended dose range. Follow the directions on your product's label.

WHEN TO TAKE

Avoid taking before bed or before exercise as the increased activity can cause heartburn or reflux.

PLEASE NOTE: *If you are on prescribed blood thinners, consult with a doctor before adding in.

OMEGA 3 FOOD SOURCES

Best fish Sources:

- Mackerel
- Salmon
- Seabass
- Oysters
- Sardines
- Shrimp
- Trout

Other Omega 3 Food Sources

- Seaweed and algae
- Chia seeds (ground or soaked for better absorption)
- Hemp Seeds
- Flax seeds (ground is best for absorption)
- Walnuts
- Edamame
- Kidney Beans

CALM MAGNESIUM (MAGNESIUM CITRATE):

Although magnesium is responsible for over 300 actions in the body, it is important to us because, it not only helps to convert your foods into usable energy, it also helps calm the nerves and balance out cortisol levels (caused by stress.) This will help your body to relax, which can help with getting deep & REM sleep. Deep sleep is important because that is the kind of sleep you need for the body to best repair, rebuild, and detoxify.

- Calm Magnesium is also beneficial when it comes to addressing bowel movement issues, and in combination with omega 3 and a probiotic, can help make significant improvements.
- The most effective Calm Magnesium is in powdered form. The pill form doesn't have the same effect.
- It comes plain or flavoured. The flavoured ones have stevia added, but the benefit outweighs the effect of stevia if it keeps you taking it regularly.
- **Make sure you are dissolving the calm mag in warm to hot water to activate the ingredients.

DOSE

1-2 tsp per day is recommended. Follow the directions on your product's label.

WHEN TO TAKE

Take at night as directed before bed. You might need to play around with the dose to find what works for you. Start with the recommended dose and increase in small increments to get the desired effect.

PLEASE NOTE: When it comes to magnesium, there are better sources than the one I suggest. However, for the purpose of weight loss, the magnesium citrate powder works best. Natural Calm Mag is a good brand but there are other mag. citrate powders available.

Also note: it is CALM Mag NOT CAL Mag.

MAGNESIUM FOOD SOURCES:

- Dark Leafy Greens spinach, kale, collard greens, Swiss chard
- Pumpkin Seeds
- Nuts especially almonds, cashews and Brazil nuts
- Tuna
- Avocados
- Bananas
- Legumes
- Whole grains

EXTRAS:

The following are a few extra add-ins that may be a benefit and worth considering.

DIGESTIVE BITTERS:

- Bitters are drops that you put into water in-between meals. Look for Canadian bitters, not Swedish. Swedish bitters can contain a mild laxative which is not recommended. Follow package directions for dose.
- If you have known digestive issues, or digestive issues that are as simple as getting bloated after eating raw veg or nuts and seeds, you may want to add in some digestive bitters.
- Digestive bitters help build up digestive enzymes that help with processing and getting nutrients from food.
- Bitters are better than taking digestive enzymes because they don't just help in the moment to process food, they also help to build up digestive enzymes that are normally created by eating raw foods.
- Bitters are also beneficial for anyone missing their gallbladder or suffering from acid reflux as they help to stimulate bile production.

DOSE

1-2 ml up to 3 times per day as directed on the label.

WHEN TO TAKE

Take between meals or 15 mins before meals.

PREBIOTIC WITH ADDED CLEAR FIBER:

- If you have inflammation, digestive, or bowel movement issues, you might want to pick up a prebiotic with added clear fiber.

- Prebiotic is food for the probiotic and together can help improve digestion and bowel movements.

- It is being used more and more in gut therapy to address things like bowel movement issues, leaky gut, high histamine levels, inflammation, insulin resistance, Crohns, and Colitis.

DOSE

Follow directions on your product's label.

WHEN TO TAKE

Prebiotic can be taken any time of day.

PREBIOTIC FOOD SOURCES

- Garlic (raw)
- Onions (raw or lightly cooked)
- Leeks
- Asparagus
- Radishes
- Bananas
- Apples
- Flaxseeds
- Cabbage
- Dandelion greens and root
- Shiitake mushrooms
- Oats, Bran, Barley
- Hemp seeds
- Unpasteurized apple cider vinegar

COLLAGEN:

- Taking collagen helps with tissue repair, improving the quality of hair and nails, but more importantly skin, which is important when it comes to weight loss.

- It's a non-essential protein naturally found in the body that depletes at a rate of 1% yearly after the age of 21.

- Because collagen is a non-essential protein it doesn't count towards protein in a meal.

- Collagen can also help with internal tissue repair and aid the body in making all the changes we are asking of it, as well as helping to maintain muscle mass.

- Most commonly sold in powder form and can be mixed into coffee, tea, water, oatmeal, yogurt etc.

- Collagen comes in either bovine sourced or marine sourced. Marine is better for skin and bovine is better for maintaining muscle mass, but both are effective. You can do your own research or speak to someone at your local health food store, to see which source and which brand is best for you.

- I personally use marine collagen. Specifically, the "Within Us TruMarine" brand and "Deep Marine" brand. But there are many quality brands to choose from.

DOSE

5-10g is the average dose recommendation. Follow the directions on your product's label.

WHEN TO TAKE

Collagen can be taken any time of day.

We will be posting a secondary supplement list in the weeks ahead with some examples of products that can amplify your results once your body is ready and you have laid a strong foundation.

Right now, you want to stick to the basics and be mindful about adding in too many things at once, which can just end up stressing the body and slowing the process.

When it comes to bowel movements specifically, we want to be mindful to allow the body to make new connections on its own without interfering too much. There is a separate Post on Bowel Movements which lists supplements that can help specifically with bowel movement issues.

TO RECAP:

SUPPLEMENTS THAT ARE KEY RIGHT NOW ARE:

- Probiotic
- Vitamin D
- Omega 3 or 3-6-9 combo
- Calm magnesium

IF YOU HAVE DIGESTIVE ISSUES CONSIDER:

- Canadian Digestive bitters
- Prebiotic

SKIN, TISSUE REPAIR, AND MAINTAIN MUSCLE MASS:

- Collagen

WHEN IT COMES TO DOSES:

- Due to the many variables based on the large variety of products and individual needs, follow as directed on the package.

WHEN TO TAKE:

- Because everyone will have different needs and some of you are taking medications and other supplements, it's best to grab a pen and paper and make some notes on what times work best, given your individual needs and situation. Check in with your pharmacist or healthcare provider to inquire about any medications that could affect the timing of supplements.

We will be chatting about the supplements all week. Watch out for the post on FAQs.

There is no rush to add these in and you don't need to start taking them all at once. You can take your time adding them in, and they can be added in at any time.

Please take time to head over to the Facebook Group and watch the quick video that accompanies this post.

**If for any reason you feel uncomfortable taking these or cannot take them for whatever reason, please understand they are simply recommended, but not necessarily make or break when it comes to weight loss. **

FAQ'S ABOUT SUPPLEMENTS

Here's a list of frequently asked questions having to do with supplements.

1. Where should I purchase the supplements?

Shopping around can save you money so be sure to check different places if you can. Your local health food store or pharmacies are great if you want to talk to someone for recommendations. Here are a few good online shopping options as well:

- Bedrugsmart.ca (Canada & US)
- Well.ca (Canada)
- Vitamart.ca (Canada)
- Vitaminshoppe.com (US)
- Thrivemarket.com (US)
- Amazon.ca and .com (Canada & US)
- COSTCO (Canada & US) also has lots of supplements at great prices.

2. If I'm taking my probiotic in the morning, should I take it before or after lemon water or acv?

You can take it before or after. Just wait about 10 minutes or so in between.

3. Can I take magnesium citrate pills?

If the powder isn't available where you live then yes, take the capsules but keep in mind they aren't as effective as the powder.

4. Can we take supplements in gummy form?

The short answer is NO. Gummies are for kids and are not as effective. They also contain artificial colour and sweeteners.

5. I take another magnesium supplement, Should I still take the calm mag?

Yes. There are hundreds of different magnesium supplements out there. The calm mag (or magnesium citrate powder) is suggested specifically to go with this program. You can continue taking your other magnesium, but we suggest you also take the Calm Mag.

6. Can collagen count as my protein for breakfast?

No, the protein in collagen is an incomplete protein. Plus, you can't drink your breakfast.

7. **When is the best time to take collagen?**

    Collagen can be taken any time of day, with or without food.

8. **I'm having acid reflux when taking the omega 3.**

    Try any or all of these things:

    - Put the capsules in the fridge or freezer.
    - Take just before a meal instead of after.
    - Switch brands or try the oil if using capsules.

9. **I take a multivitamin. Can I take that instead?**

    You can continue to take any other supplements you were taking prior to the program but not in place of the ones recommended here.

LET'S TALK BOWEL MOVEMENTS

If you have always suffered from bowel movement issues, then rest assured you will see significant improvement by following the program.

During this Process, because we piggyback the body's natural detox response, your bowel movements will be all over the place, meaning every shape, size and consistency.

You may experience bouts of constipation, which are normal before detox or when the body is focused on making changes. You may also experience episodes of diarrhea or loose bowel movements, which are a normal occurrence when the body is in active "detox" or eating any foods your body may be sensitive to.

Your digestive health is directly associated with, and affects your bowel movements. Food goes in and the byproduct eventually needs to make its way out. So, if you have experienced constipation issues in the past, this could have played a major role in your body feeling the need to store fat.

Here is what you can do, above and beyond following The Program, to help improve your bowel movements:

LET'S TALK CONSTIPATION:

THE BASICS:

- Drink lots of water

- Be sure to add leafy greens to meals

- Add in, and regularly take, the basic supplements: Omega 3, Vit D, Probiotic, and Calm magnesium.

In addition to what is listed above in regards to the basics, which all work together on Plan, we also suggest looking into adding:

1. **PREBIOTIC:**

- Prebiotic is food for your probiotic. Prebiotic does come in pill form but is best to get in a clear fiber.

- You can also increase your intake of prebiotic foods that help with digestion like: Onions, garlic, leeks, chickpeas, lentils, kidney beans, bananas, grapefruit, bran, barley, and oats.

2. **DIGESTIVE BITTERS:**

- Digestive bitters are herbs that support digestive function by stimulating bitter receptors on the tongue, stomach, gallbladder, and pancreas.

- They work to promote digestive juices such as stomach acid, bile, and enzymes, which help to break down food and assist in the absorption of nutrients.
- Look for Canadian bitters that come in drops you add to water.
- Take bitters about 20 minutes before a meal to signal your body to produce more saliva, bile, and stomach acid.

3. **VITAMIN C:**
- When taking higher doses of vitamin C, the extra or un-absorbed vitamin C pulls water into your intestines, which can help soften your stool.
- Take 30 mins before food in the morning, dose is dependent on the individual and can range from 90-2000 mg.

4. **B COMPLEX:**
- B 12, B 1 & B 5 deficiency can cause constipation. If your constipation is caused by low levels of B's, increasing your daily intake of this nutrient may help ease your symptoms.
- B 12 or B complex is part of the secondary supplements list I will be sending out in a few weeks.
- Not essential to weight loss, but it is key in supporting metabolic function, which can significantly help with weight loss, by helping to improve your energy.
- You may prefer to eat more foods rich in this vitamin rather than take a supplement.

EXAMPLES OF FOODS RICH IN B VITAMINS INCLUDE:
- Meat (red meat, poultry, fish)
- Beef
- Liver
- Trout
- Salmon
- Tuna fish
- Whole grains (brown rice, barley, millet)
- Eggs and dairy products (milk, cheese)
- Legumes (beans, lentils)
- Seeds and nuts (sunflower seeds, almonds)
- Dark, leafy vegetables (broccoli, spinach)
- Fruits (citrus fruits, avocados, bananas)

5.   **TRIPHALA:**

- Used in Ayurvedic medicine for thousands of years. It's thought to support bowel health and aid digestion. As an antioxidant, it's also thought to detoxify the body and support the immune system.

- Triphala helps to keep the stomach, small intestine and large intestine healthy by flushing out toxins from the body.

- Triphala is available in supplement form, as a pill, and in powder form. The powder is meant to be dissolved in warm water and consumed as tea. It can taste bitter but can be mixed with honey or lemon without diminishing its effects.

- Triphala supplements have varying daily dosages based upon the manufacturer. It's important to follow package directions exactly.

- Triphala may be most effective when taken right before bed with a large glass of warm water.

- Some people prefer to take this supplement on an empty stomach, while others prefer to take it with food. Discuss these options with your doctor.

6.   **EXERCISE/MOVE YOUR BODY:**

- Exercise helps constipation by lowering the time it takes food to move through the large intestine. This limits the amount of water your body absorbs from the stool.

- Cardio exercise speeds up your breathing and heart rate, helping to stimulate the natural squeezing of muscles in your intestines which helps to move stool out quickly.

- Something as simple as going for a walk after dinner can make all the difference when it comes to improving digestion.

7.   **TIME AND CONSISTENCY:**

- It is important to note that in most cases the body just needs time to rewire how it has come to function over the years.

- The foods you are eating, and the overall structure of The Program will help from a baseline level to address constipation issues.

- Try to keep things routine and be patient with the process, but also don't suffer. Sometimes you need to take something stronger like an over-the-counter laxative to help the body work through any backlog.

LET'S TALK LOOSE BOWEL MOVEMENTS:

Loose bowel movements can be unnerving but also a normal part of the process due to all the water you are drinking, leafy greens you are eating, as well as fiber rich foods like fruit and veggies which all contribute to a natural daily detox.

In most cases, it's nothing to be concerned about. However, here are some things you can do to address:

1. Continuing to focus on digestive health. It can be a great idea to add in the prebiotic and bitters to help strengthen your digestive system.

2. Keep a journal and record how you are feeling after eating meals and snacks as sometimes food sensitivities can pop up that can cause loose BM and discomfort.

3. Dairy and gluten are the most common sensitivities, but it can come down to specific food choices like a kind of fruit for example, or even spicy food.

4. Decrease calm magnesium. Although the calm mag is rarely the sole issue for loose BM, decreasing it slightly may help.

5. If you are concerned about nutrient loss, rest assured, it's not a major concern when following the plan.

6. You can add trace minerals to your water or add in a pinch of pink rock salt or Celtic salt to your warm water and lemon in the morning and/or water throughout the day.

7. Add in Psyllium fiber. You never want to add in fiber while constipated as it can sometimes make the situation worse. It is however an excellent time to add in if experiencing loose bowel movements.

Psyllium is non-dependent and when added in, attaches itself to toxins stored in your fat cells and helps to draw them out. This can help make your bowel movements more binding and effective for fat loss.

- The soluble fiber also helps lower blood cholesterol levels and control blood sugar levels. You can also get this type of fiber from oats, barley, oranges, dried beans and lentils.
- Comes in pill or powder form. I personally like the pills.
- Take before bed or in between meals.

TO RECAP:

The body will be working hard to address digestive and BM issues. Given enough time, your body will aim to make significant improvements.

Although usually nothing to be concerned about, when it comes to BM issues, it is always recommended to check in with your doctor.

Some conditions including Crohn's disease, celiac disease, IBS, thyroid issues and medications can be the cause of loose BM, but if your changes in BM go hand in hand with following the program, chances are there is nothing to be concerned about and given the time, the body will sort out and address it on its own.

Please take time to head over to the Facebook Group and watch the quick video that accompanies this post.

IS IT A FRUIT OR VEG?

This question gets asked a lot. Especially in relation to tomatoes and avocados. Because they are technically fruits, we get asked if they can be eaten at fruit snack, but on this program, we classify tomatoes as a veg and avocado as a healthy fat.

DID YOU KNOW....

A fruit develops from a flower and produces seeds or a pit. Like a tomato... and many other fruits we think of as vegetables inside and out of this program.

In the botanical world, the word "vegetable" doesn't even exist. What we call vegetables they refer to as leaves, stems, roots, flower buds etc. Like celery is a stem and radishes are roots.

The word "vegetable" is only a culinary term.

There are many foods on plan that are technically fruits, but we use them as veg. And there are some fruits that we categorize as healthy fats.

LET'S BREAK IT DOWN...

TECHNICALLY FRUITS BUT WE USE THEM AS VEGETABLES ON PLAN:

- Tomatoes
- Cucumbers
- Peppers
- Peas
- Green beans
- Eggplant
- Okra
- Corn
- Zucchini
- Olives
- Pumpkin
- Squash

NOTE: Even though these are technically fruits, we use them as vegetables on plan. Then there are fruits (technically) that we use as fats on plan.

TECHNICALLY FRUITS BUT WE USE AS HEALTHY FATS ON PLAN

- Avocado

- Nuts

- Olives (to confuse matters more, this is also a vegetable on plan)

- Coconut (technically a fruit, a nut, and a seed!) But we use it as a healthy fat on plan.

Watermelon is both a fruit and a vegetable, but we use it as a fruit on plan and did you know that rhubarb is actually a vegetable? (Remember the stem example I used with the celery above? Same, same).

Are you confused yet?!

We could go down a scientific rabbit hole with this subject but just wanted to provide some clarity as well as some fun facts!

LET'S TALK OILS

It's important to choose the right oil for the right job. Oils are used in all kinds of things from dressings to marinades, sautéing, searing, stir frying, roasting etc. But not all oils are created equal.

When it comes to cooking with oils, things can easily get complicated. Levels of saturation, smoke points, cold pressed, unrefined, hydrogenated…. blah blah blah. It's easy to go down a rabbit hole when it comes to oils, so I'm going to try and simplify things a bit.

I'm going to break down some of those terms I mentioned above so you know what to keep in mind when choosing your oils

SMOKE POINT:

The point at which an oil starts to smoke when heated is it's smoke point. You want to avoid letting oils get to the smoke point because it indicates that the oil has been damaged and is releasing harmful chemicals into the air by way of smoke. If you accidentally bring oil to its smoking point, toss it out and start again at a lower temperature. PRO TIPS: Heat the pan first and then add your oil, let it heat for a few seconds then add your ingredients. This can prevent the oil from ever reaching its smoke point. In most cases for frying and sautéing high heat isn't necessary. Even for searing meats, a medium high heat works just great!

COMMON OILS WITH A HIGHER SMOKE POINT:

Refined olive, avocado, coconut, canola, grapeseed, peanut oil, sunflower, safflower and sesame.

REFINED VS UNREFINED:

Unrefined oils are only lightly filtered and have better flavour, colour, and fragrance than refined oils. The bottle will say "unrefined" or "cold pressed" They are more nutritious and are best used unheated as in a salad dressing or very low heat cooking. All the healthy stuff will disappear if heated too much.

COMMON UNREFINED OILS:

Extra virgin olive, avocado, coconut, nut oils such as walnut and almond, sesame oil. Extra virgin olive oil may not say "cold pressed" or "unrefined" because "extra virgin" means the same thing.

Naturally refined oils are more finely filtered with the use of a little heat. This can reduce the nutrient level and flavour but also makes them more resistant to smoking. They are not chemically refined like large crop oils (see below) Many common ones listed above under "Smoke Point".

WHAT ABOUT BUTTER?

Butter is great for cooking and has a medium smoke point so keep the heat to medium temperatures when using it for cooking. Ghee or clarified butter has a higher smoke point so can be used for higher temperature cooking.

Organic butter is always best, if your budget allows.

WHAT TO AVOID:

Unfortunately, many of the oils found on the shelves in the grocery store are chemically processed and are produced in large crops that are heavily sprayed with chemical pesticides. Oils like canola, safflower, soy, corn, palm, sunflower...as well as the generically labeled "vegetable oils" (which is just a combination of any of the above listed oils). These often contain trans fats as well. They are best to avoid or use sparingly.

HYDROGENATED OILS:

This is a highly chemical process that converts a naturally liquid oil into a solid oil. Best to avoid these or products containing these oils. Shortening and margarine are hydrogenated oils although there are now many non-hydrogenated margarines on the market so check those labels!

SO NOW WHAT?

When shopping for oils, look at the labels for words like "refined" "unrefined", "cold pressed", "extra virgin" and "organic".

LAST BUT NOT LEAST... Nothing to worry or stress about from a weight loss perspective. You don't need to throw out any oils you don't think are good. We are just looking to provide you with some more information to continue making good choices when at the grocery store.

LET'S TALK DOUBLE DETOX & YOUR MENSTRUATION CYCLE

As much of a pain as it can be, your period is an awesome opportunity to capitalize on fat loss each month!

Because My Method of weight loss uses the same detox process that the body uses when you are sick (cold or flu), have food poisoning, or when you have your period, we can use those times to help with the weight loss process.

Which is where the concept of double detox comes from.

Your period each month is a time where the body looks to reset, to balance hormones, and to get rid of any fat it doesn't need.

When your MENSTRUAL CYCLE hits:

- Be consistent with supplements
- Increase the calm magnesium

Magnesium contributes to energy production, helps with digestion, relieves anxiety to name a few, but it can also help relieve PMS symptoms and keep your hormones more balanced. Taking magnesium daily has been proven effective in preventing menstrual migraines as your magnesium levels tend to be a lot lower on your period due to your hormones.

Magnesium is also effective in relaxing muscles, which can help with any cramping.

Magnesium can also help boost your mood by playing a role in serotonin production. Serotonin is a mood-boosting hormone. You can add an extra dose during the day or increase your dose at night. Taking during the day won't cause drowsiness as your body isn't producing Melatonin at that time.

Be mindful of iron issues. When blood is lost every month, the iron in red blood cells is also lost. If your monthly iron intake and absorption does not replace the iron lost during your period, you can end up with iron deficiency, which affects not only your energy, but your ability to lose weight.

(**If you think you might be low in Iron, be sure to check in with your doctor**).

Here are some tips to help support the body during Double Detox:

- Extra water
- Hit all meals and snacks
- Keep portions on the smaller side to allow the body to stay focused on the task at hand
- Lighter on the carbs and heavier on the leafy greens at lunch and dinner for increased roughage to help keep moving things in and out

- Eat as early as possible
- Go to bed earlier to help the body get extra rest
- Take warm epsom salt baths

The intention here is to help the body stay focused on the task at hand and capitalize on the natural detox process.

It's also key to note that this process allows the body the opportunity to balance hormones, which can lead to cycle syncing. Cycle syncing is the practice of eating, exercising, and aligning your lifestyle choices according to your menstrual cycle.

Cycle syncing is something that happens naturally while following the plan because of the holistic approach we are taking to lose weight.

This is why it's normal for your period to come early, late, or look and feel different than what you are used to while following the plan. Although this can be unnerving, rest assured your body is doing what's best to allow your body to work at optimal levels.

And as always, if ever you feel something is more off than it should be, always check in with your doctor.

Please take time to head over to the Facebook Group and watch the quick video that accompanies this post.

WEEK 3 GUIDELINES: CONSISTENCY & MINDFULNESS

This week has us discussing issues and associations when it comes to food. The goal is to be as consistent as possible to allow the body time to calm down and get used to the changes you have already made. This is also where we start to address portions. How are your portions? How do you feel while eating? How do you know when you're full? What are your habits & hang-ups? How is your body responding?

LET'S TALK CONSISTENCY

I would love to tell you this is where things start to get exciting, but the goal of Week 3 is actually quite the opposite.

Week 2 had you working on fine tuning and perfecting the changes that you have made so far, as well as the addition of the bonus snacks and supplements.

Moving into Week 3, the goal is to be as consistent as possible to allow the body time to calm down and adjust from the changes you have made in the past few weeks. Follow the food plan, make nutrient rich choices, continue to eat to satisfaction, add in any supplements, and work the water.

If you are continually feeling unsatisfied at the end of the day, or hungry to the point where it's distracting during the day, be sure to add in the bonus snack/s when needed.

Consistency is key as we are still in the phase of making the body feel confident that it no longer needs the stored fat it has been hanging onto for whatever reason; high stress, lack of sleep, long periods of time without eating, just to name a few.

I recognize this is not the most exciting week, but it is a very important one. It is essential that you establish routine within the body to lay a strong foundation we can work with.

The first few weeks of the program were about giving the body what it needs so as you move forward, you can manipulate it into focusing more on what you want it to do, which is to drop fat.

If you are starting to feel bored with the routine or the foods you are eating, rest assured, that is normal for where we are in the process. Rather than looking for alternatives or swapping recipes to make things more exciting, I want you to indulge in the boredom.

If you are not bored, that is OK too, as some people enjoy the routine.

This week is key for these reasons:

- It is important to continue to allow the body to adjust to the changes you have made in the first few weeks so it can calm down internally and focus less on digestion and inflammation and more on making change.

- If you have ever used food for anything other than nutritional requirements, like eating out of boredom, distraction, stress, reward and so on, this stage will address that.

- This week helps you get more in tune with your body's needs over your wants.

- This week also allows the body time to adjust its hunger levels, which will have you feeling fuller faster as your portions naturally decrease.

At the end of this week, things will start to come together for you as your body starts to change, weight starts to drop, and you get to a place where you feel so good that the process becomes about maintaining that feeling and building on it as we move forward.

LET'S TALK MINDFULNESS

This is when we start to focus on fat loss by focusing on maximizing the food plan and being even more in tune to your portion sizes.

Because we don't weigh, measure or count anything when it comes to portions, the first step to adjusting them is to put some time into increasing the mind-body connection even further, by paying attention to how the body is responding to your meals and snacks.

It sounds a bit corny, but there is a reason why people always talk about the mind-body connection.

Most people, when asked what makes them stop eating or how they know when they are satisfied, will tell you it's when they are done eating everything on their plate or until they feel full. And because most people have been eating until they feel physically full, they end up eating way more food than they need. And then they get used to eating more than they need, which then becomes the norm.

**The goal is to get to a place where your body tells you very clearly WHEN to eat, WHAT to eat, and HOW MUCH to eat. **

The process of weighing and measuring foods, counting calories and macros is not a normal way to eat. Neither is this food plan formula of eating I currently have you following.

So it's important to note, as we move forward in the program, we are going to transition into more of a natural way of eating. But first, we need to make sure you are completely in tune with where you are now. Which brings us to the purpose of mindfulness, where the focus is on addressing portions by being mindful about how your body is responding before, during, and after you eat.

HERE IS WHAT YOU ARE TO DO:

ASK YOURSELF THESE 4 QUESTIONS

1. **Before you eat, ask yourself if you are even hungry:**

    *   The goal is to bring awareness to your changing hunger levels. For example, sometimes you are really hungry but then when you eat, you get full fast. Other times you are not hungry at all, but when you start to eat, you feel hungry. Both are normal and you are still to eat all meals and snacks regardless of hunger levels.

2. **When serving or portioning out your food and before you eat...ask yourself:**

    *   How is this portion for me?
    *   How would I feel if I ate all of this?
    *   You may not get a really strong response or any answer from your body at first, but trust that after a few days of talking to yourself, your body will start to talk back.

3. **While eating your food, pay attention to how you feel and ask yourself:**

    *   Are you getting full, is this food satisfying you?
    *   How would you feel if you took a few more bites?
    *   How would you feel if you stop eating now?
    *   Do you feel any physical effects of eating?

4. **When you are done eating, ask yourself how you feel:**

    *   Do you feel full and if so, what is your definition of full?
    *   How do you know when you have eaten enough?
    *   How do you feel physically? Meaning, is it a physically full belly feeling or is it more of an insulin rush or a tired feeling? Or is it that you just eat everything on your plate because it's there kind of thing? Or maybe you feel like you could eat more?

I know some of you may be inclined to start cutting and decreasing portions thinking it's going to get you ahead. I promise you it won't. It will only lead to confusion down the road if you miss this very important step.

If you follow these simple steps, your portions will naturally decrease on their own. For now, focus on eating enough food so that when you are done and walk away from your food, you don't feel any physical effects. Meaning, when you walk away from your food you shouldn't physically feel like you ate. If you do, chances are you have eaten too much.

**With that said...You are NOT TRYING to decrease portions sizes based on counting, weighing, measuring, or what they look like. **

This is about being in tune to them. Your hunger levels will change day to day so **it's about what the portions FEEL like... not what they LOOK like**, so each day might look different, portion size wise. If you decrease portions by too much too soon, you will have a hard time moving forward in the Program.

This week is about being more in tune with your body's needs so when we do start to address portions, you will know what to do. Although you may notice your portions are naturally getting smaller, make sure to still eat to satisfaction regardless of what that portion looks like day to day.

TO RECAP:

Your task for this week is a very simple but important one: to be as consistent as possible and to take time to connect with your body and get in the habit of being mindful of hunger levels and portions.

Ask yourself the 4 Questions. Try to eat without distractions so you can focus on your body's signals.

As we move forward in the coming weeks, you will need to have a clear understanding of when you are hungry, what you are hungry for, and how much.

As a look ahead into Week 4, we will start to reduce portion sizes so it is very important that it comes off the heels of your body feeling satisfied and confident that it no longer needs the fat it has been storing and holding on to.

CONSISTENCY REMAINS KEY.

This is a very exciting time. You have patiently been putting in the time and work to lay a super strong foundation that will not only lead to weight loss success but will set you up to move forward from this process to live a normal life when it comes to food.

The goal is to not only lose weight and lose it in a way that is sustainable, but also to move on from the fight of constantly trying to lose. To let go of the "diet talk", the counting, weighing, measuring and stress from trying to lose over the years.

Let's work on changing that internal dialog this week while also being mindful of your portions and maximizing your efforts each day.

Please take time to head over to the Facebook Group and watch the quick video that accompanies this post.

WHY MINDFULNESS IS KEY

I know a lot of you have probably read over the Week 3 Guidelines and are left thinking "what the heck?!" You might be also thinking "I'm not really into all this mindfulness and meditation hullabaloo so this just isn't really for me". I get that but let me explain why, especially when it comes to weight loss; it's super important and you don't want to just blow it off.

When it comes to weight loss, there is never enough emphasis put on the mind-body connection. Especially in Western societies where large (HUGE!) portions have become the norm. Many of us were brought up being taught to not waste food and finish everything on the plate, sometimes not even being allowed to leave the table until everything was finished. "After all there are starving children in Africa!" How many of you heard that growing up?

This idea that you must clean your plate goes way back in history and has to do with food shortages beginning in World War I. It has become totally normal for parents to urge their kids to finish everything on their plates, regardless of how they feel. So, at a very young age we start learning how NOT to listen to our bodies. We have literally been trained to be mindless eaters, blindly shoveling food in until the plate is clean and that "oh-so-glorious" insulin rush comes in from overeating. Anything sounding familiar?

So that brings us to why this week is so important. We need to take the time to unlearn all of that training and start to feel and understand what our bodies are telling us. It's not going to be easy. For many, it's been basically your entire life being taught not to listen. It's not easy or quick to unlearn and retrain this way of thinking...or not thinking in this case.

Start slow and don't expect to get it right away. You may not have any answers to those questions when you first start and that's okay. You might say "I never feel hungry." That's probably because you have spent years going very long periods of time without eating. Keep asking and you will begin to have answers. It will take time and lots and lots of practice. Just like learning a new skill, you need repetition, and it will slowly become more natural. This isn't a week you are trying to nail as it is not as straightforward as just following the Food Formula. We are asking you to dig a bit deeper here.

Take the time to:

- Focus
- Slow down
- Pay attention

In my experience, learning to listen to your body's cues, especially when it comes to portion sizes, is THE MOST IMPORTANT PART OF THIS PROGRAM. It's the thing that will keep that weight off. For good! You will always be in tune and very aware when you've let yourself go off track and your body will let you know…. if you are listening.

MY TOP TIPS FOR NAVIGATING MINDFULNESS:

TRY NOT TO EAT WHILE DISTRACTED

Watching television, your phone, driving etc. can take the focus away from connecting with your body signals so try to eat in a calm state away from rushing and distractions where you can slow down and pay attention. If you are eating with a distraction, be extra diligent about checking in with yourself periodically about how you are feeling.

EAT WHAT'S MOST APPEALING ON YOUR PLATE

You still want to prepare your meals using the guidelines of more veg at lunch and more protein at dinner but don't put too much focus on that while eating and being mindful. Instead, eat what's most appealing to you in the moment (more mindfulness) and don't worry if you think you had more protein at lunch or less at dinner.

AM I STILL HUNGRY?

"Eating to satisfaction" can be a hard concept to grasp at first, so try rewording it into something else. "Am I still hungry" "Is my body wanting more or is it my mind or my taste buds wanting more?". Come up with your own question that is easier for you to connect with if you need.

WAIT A FEW MINUTES

If you decide you are satisfied but just can't believe all the food left on your plate, wait 10 minutes or so and if you decide you need a few more bites then have them. You will often find that you don't.

TRY NOT TO BE "AFRAID"

It's normal to feel anxious about being hungry later because you think you didn't eat enough. Remember that the next snack or meal is right around the corner and you can also add in bonus snacks if you need them.

SAVE FOOD FOR LATER

Remember that when you don't finish what's on your plate you can always save it for later.

LET'S TALK GROUP CHECKLIST

As we move forward the conversation is going to be more forward moving...it's a good time to make sure you are up to speed on the basics.

Even though we switch up the Food Formula as we go through the 12 weeks, nailing the basics sooner than later is key, so that as we move forward, you are ready for each new week.

Be sure to review the basics so your path moving forward is as clear and calm as possible.

Here are some tips on how to navigate and keep up with the information in the Group:

1. **EMAILS**

   - Please note, we are not emailing out any information as everything is posted in the Facebook Support Group and can be found in Guides and Topics.

2. **CHECK INTO THE SUPPORT GROUP DAILY**

   - Be sure to use the GUIDES section to keep track of anything new being posted each day.

   - Most of the information in this Workbook has an accompanying video posted in the Group. Be sure to check into the group and watch all the videos as they can provide additional information and clarity.

   - Be sure to use the Topics buttons to review any previous posts.

   - And be sure to use the magnifying glass search at the top to search all posts on any topic. Make sure you are searching in the Group and not all of Facebook.

3. **WATCH THE DAILY CHECK IN VIDEO**

   - This is a short daily video where I check in and let you know what you need to know or focus on each day.

   - These are key as I talk in more detail on what you need to know each day and will become more instructional as we go.

4. **ASK YOUR QUESTIONS ON THE DAILY QUESTIONS POST**

   - The questions post is always pinned to the top of the page.

   - This is where you are to ask any questions you have. Ask as many as you need to be clear about the process.

   - Keep in mind, we are asking you to base those questions on the information you have already reviewed.

5. WE KINDLY ASK YOU REFRAIN FROM SENDING US PERSONAL DM'S AND EMAILS

- Once the group is up and running, it is our primary focus. Asking questions in the group is the quickest way to get an answer.

- You signed up to participate in the group format, so questions are to be asked in the group.

6. WATCH ANY ADDITIONAL SUPPORT VIDEOS

- Each day, I will be posting info relevant to The Process that you will need to know. We are expecting people to keep up with new information. The videos are just as important as the written posts, so be sure to read the post as well as watch the video.

- We are mindful of your time, but also mindful of the info you need to be successful.

7. WATCH FACEBOOK LIVE

- Weekdays from 9 10am, Monday to Thursday from 7 8pm and Saturday from 10 11am EST, unless otherwise noted.

- This is a live Q and A format. Gina answers as many questions as possible in the hour.

- Although this is suggested, watching the Lives is not required...they can be of great value, help give greater insight into the process, as well as hearing input from previous members.

If you have not watched them yet, please take time to check out these 5 videos found in the Facebook Group:

1. MY METHOD
2. THE FOOD PLAN
3. DETOX
4. THE SCALE
5. WEIGHT LOSS

LET'S TALK MAXIMIZING AND 20 QUESTIONS YOU CAN ASK YOURSELF

Are you trying to figure out why you might not be losing as much or as fast as you like...then this post is for you!

Even though it is still WAY too early in The Program to be concerned about the scale, as you move forward you may find yourself wondering or questioning if you are doing everything right or if there is anything more you can do to help the process.

These are some of the questions that I will ask you...if you ask me why things are not working the way you think they should. I suggest you grab some paper and a pen and go through it making notes on the areas that need your attention.

20 QUESTIONS TO ASK YOURSELF:

1. **Are you doing everything you can to create the ideal environment for your body to focus on fat loss?**

Are you following the program 100% day in and day out? Like actually, because there is a difference between trying and doing.

- Are you being as consistent as possible, day in and day out?
- Have you watched these videos that break down the rhyme & reason behind the order of the meals and snacks? 1. My Method 2. The Food Plan 3. Let's Talk Detox 4. Let's Talk The Scale Let's Talk Weight Loss.
- Have you been as consistent as possible, this means day in and day out?
- Are you making all the necessary tweaks and changes along the way?

We are not talking about kind of, or sort of doing, we are talking about maximizing what you are doing to your full potential. Literally doing all of the things you can and need to do to be as successful as possible!

2. **Has your body had time to consistently focus on fat loss?**

- Meaning has your body had days and weeks of working the plan where nothing trumps the body from focusing on fat loss? Day in and day out? Or have you had some off days and/or off weekends?

Be real about the time your body has had to focus on fat loss. Have you been hit or miss with following the food plan, sick or stressed out, or are there things you are dealing with physically or mentally that need to be taken into account?

3. **Have you had the flu or a cold or any other sickness that your body is dealing with, or had to deal with and focus on?**

- Is your body more focused on healing right now?
- Are you taking antibiotics or meds that might mess with digestion or make you dehydrated that you need to address?
- Are you following the Sickness Protocol?

Are you following the sickness protocol and helping the body heal so it can better focus on fat loss when the time comes?

4. Are you managing your stress levels?

- Are you meditating, deep breathing, stretching, moving your body, going for walks, taking epsom salt baths and so on...and if so for how long and how often?
- Have you read the post on managing stress?

Are you really doing all you can do to help the body manage your stress? Stress can play a major role in preventing the body from focusing on fat loss. Managing your stress can go a long way in getting the scale to move.

5. Are you getting lots of deep & REM sleep?

- Are you helping your body prepare for sleep by eating earlier in the evening, going to bed earlier, keeping lights low and avoiding stimulants like TV and phone, taking a relaxing bath, keeping a journal by your bed?
- Have you read the post on Sleep?

Are you actually making changes? Or still staying up late?

6. Are you drinking enough water?

- Not just a set amount, but adjusting it according to the body's demands? (Not just "more than before" or "lots" ...are you drinking enough, spreading it out and sipping on it for maximum absorption & utilization?)
- Are you adding in salt, sole water or trace minerals?
- Have you read all of the posts on water?

7. Are you making your food as nutrient rich as possible?

- Are you adding different elements to your meals? Veg, protein, greens, healthy fats? (Not just grabbing what's convenient or easy or what you like or love...think most bang for your buck and maximum value).
- Have you read the Making Your Meals Nutrient Rich Post?

8. Are you exercising? Are you moving your body?

- If so, what are you doing and how often? Are you getting your heart rate up?

- Are you making an effort to be more active?
- Are you taking the stairs, parking further away, participating and not just sitting on the sidelines?
- Are you factoring in time for the body to repair and rebuild any damage from your workouts?
- Have you read the post on exercise?
- Are you being mindful to move?

9. **Are you helping the body while in detox?**
- Watching portions, keeping food light, drinking lots of water, eating early at night and getting lots of sleep and maximizing everything else you can and need to do?
- Have you watched the Detox Video? Have you made an effort to really understand and help the body maximize when it's in detox?

10. **Are you taking medications or have health issues that need to be factored in?**
- You can lose weight regardless of your health issues but they will impact your journey, so if there are things you can do to help the body adjust to medications and help to address or heal the issue ...it will help when it comes to the scale.
- Have you looked into other ways you can help your body heal or deal with your health issues?

11. **Are you missing any organs?**
- Are you helping the body compensate for missing organs like adding in the bile salts or digestive bitters if missing your gallbladder?
- Are you going the extra mile to help your body manage any deficiencies?

12. **Do you have hormone issues you need to address? Or that needs to be factored in?**
- Are you seeing a specialist or adding in supplements that can help?
- Have you looked into addressing hormonal issues you may be dealing with?

13. **Have you had your blood work done?**
- Do you have any deficiencies that could be affecting your body's ability to function properly?
- Have you seen or checked in with your doctor recently?
- Had a physical done?
- Are you keeping up with appointments like your Chiropractor or Therapist?

14. **Are you taking all the supplements and taking them consistently?**
- They all work together and are all key in weight loss. Are you maximizing your efforts by adding them in?

- Are you consistent with taking them?
- Have you read all the posts on supplements?

15. **Is your body changing? Has your body been focusing on repairing and rebuilding and making change?**

- What changes have you seen that can't be seen on the scale and is your body changing shape and size?
- What are the non-scale victories you are experiencing?

**Pay attention to what your body is focused on and when, the non-scale victories can be just as key because your body is always working and it can't all be about weight loss. **

16. **Are you eating a lot of red meat and meat in general or are you switching between veg proteins, seafood, fish, and meat?**

- Be mindful about those quality protein choices.
- Are you making an effort to maximize your food choices?
- Are you choosing the best options or are you stuck on eating what you like and love?

17. **Do you have any digestive issues?**

- Have you added in the supplements to help?
- Are you maximizing your food choices to help your body better digest and process your food?
- Are you eating things you are sensitive to like dairy or gluten?
- Are you keeping a journal and taking notes on how your body is responding to your food choices?

18. **Do you have issues with bowel movements and if so, what are you doing to address them?**

- Have you added in the supplements to help and are you Maximizing your food choices?
- Are you making the best choices possible?
- Are you adding leafy greens to your meals and mindful to add in fiber rich foods?

19. **Are you sabotaging yourself?**

- Do you continue to get in your own way of reaching your goals?
- Are you making choices that take you further away, not closer to, your goals?
- Are you indulging in your frustration?
- Are you having real conversations with yourself?

20. **Do you genuinely believe you have what it takes to follow through and finish?**

- Do you have faith that you can lose the weight?
- What is your WHY? What is motivating you to keep showing up and following through till the end?
- Do you truly see yourself still here at the end?

HOW TO USE THE 20 QUESTIONS AS A TOOL:

These are the questions I ask people when they say things are not working or they ask me why or what else they can do to speed things up. I suggest you take these 20 questions and give yourself a grade or a mark out of 10.

For example, when it comes to water, how are you doing on a scale of 1-10?

Or, when it comes to trying to get a better sleep, how are you doing on a scale of 1-10? Or, on a scale of 1-10, how are you doing with being consistent?

You get the idea!

Give yourself a score out of 10 and if you don't score a 10, make a list of the things that you can do that can help you address those areas and maximize your efforts.

That way you can easily see the areas that need your attention and better focus on the things you need to step up your game.

PLEASE NOTE:

If you are struggling and wondering if you are missing something along the way, these questions will help you get to the bottom of it and figure it out.

With that said, sometimes you CAN be doing everything right and all the body needs is time...but this is a good checklist to make sure.

As we continue to move forward in the program and the focus becomes more about getting the body to focus specifically on fat loss, it is key that you maximize your efforts far beyond the food, water and supplements.

As you can see, there are a variety of factors that may be affecting how your body is responding along the way.

Being realistic about those factors will help you make the adjustments you need to keep moving forward so you can successfully lose as much weight as possible in the time frame we have.

MAXIMIZING YOUR FOOD CHOICES

In the first few weeks of The Program, we really want the focus to be on settling into the routine. We want you to nail the Basic Food Formula so moving forward you are super clear, since it is the basis of the whole Program. Now is the time where you can start leveling up your efforts by maximizing everything you are doing, including your food choices.

I'm going to give you some things to think about tweaking as we move along. Keep in mind these are things that some people never have issues with and can continue to see results without having to think about, reduce, or eliminate. You have to decide for yourself how relaxed or hard core you want to be.

This is also a post you might decide to revisit down the road, after we start focusing on fat loss, if the scale seems to be stuck or moving slowly. Sometimes the smallest tweaks can make all the difference.

If you want to be really hard core (like I was) here are some things to keep in mind around your food choices. Remember it's also okay to decide you want to take a more relaxed approach and aren't in that much of a hurry. But for those of you who want to see that scale move as much as possible in the time that we have, then Maximizing is what you want to be doing.

Here are some questions to ask yourself. Places where you might be able to make some tweaks and move on to the next phase of leveling up and Maximizing your efforts.

1.   Are You Still Eating Bread?

I can honestly say that I didn't eat a single piece of bread while I was losing weight ...Okay maybe a bit of baguette, once I was close to the end but not until then. I used to eat bread every day, especially with my eggs at breakfast, and honestly didn't know if I could go without it. I mean who eats eggs without toast? Although, when asked if you can have bread, Gina always says you "can", but she also always follows it with "but it can slow down the process". That was my reason right there to stop eating it. And guess what? I never missed it. That's the truth. And even now that I can have it, I rarely do. When I do, I really enjoy it, but most of the time I have no desire for it.

Here's the thing about bread...by following this plan we are trying to decrease the amount of insulin your body is using which will eventually help you feel more satisfied with smaller portions. Things like bread and pasta require a lot of insulin to break down, no matter what it's made of. It's the process of making it that has it turn to sugar too quickly which can affect blood sugar levels. What about crackers? Crackers are the same as bread. There is nothing in them that your body needs. They, like bread, are just a transport vessel, or a way to add some crunch. So, if you really want to maximize, I would skip the crackers.

2.   Are You Eating Popcorn or Snacking At Night?

We know it can take some of you a bit longer to make the changes you need to make to address your cravings, and no doubt many of you are still working on that. Popcorn was added in the beginning to help with that transition. Since then, we have talked about hunger and how to address it. Be sure to watch the Hunger Video if you haven't already. We have also talked about how the body doesn't need food after dark and how eating and snacking can mess with your sleep and prevent your body from doing the work it needs to do during sleep. So now that you understand that, it's time to cut the popcorn or any night time snacking. It absolutely will slow down the process if you continue to snack at night.

3.   Are You Still Having Heavier Carbs At Dinner?

I know we all love our potatoes and rice at dinner time, but the body absolutely does not need these heavier carbs (energy foods) at night. Unless you do heavy workouts or play sports at night you should seriously think about cutting out those heavier carbs at dinner. Add them to your lunch instead when you feel you need them.

4.   Are You Eating Breakfast?

Or have you been purposefully skipping it because you are thinking less food (or calories) is going to get you ahead? Or maybe you just aren't making an effort to be organized and have something easy to grab if you are busy. Make no mistake, having a protein packed breakfast will absolutely help with the weight loss process. Although it is fine to skip it, and sometimes it's just going to happen, it will help with the process if you have it. Even if it's just one egg or a couple bites of chicken or a few spoonfuls of yogurt with hemp hearts.

5.   Is Your Breakfast Truly Protein Rich?

When eating oatmeal, cereals, or yogurt with added sugar and/or fruit for breakfast are you making sure that protein is the star of the show? The more sugar and carbs in your breakfast the more protein and fat you need to counteract that. Be sure you are bumping up the protein as much as you can. Remember to choose foods that give you the most bang for your buck.

6.   How's Your Sugar Adding Up?

Let's talk about sugar for a minute. Yes, we do say that it's perfectly fine to have it in your coffee or tea, on your oatmeal or yogurt, and also okay if you buy yogurt which already contains sugar. But ask yourself this: Am I having sweetened yogurt, then adding fruit to it and also having several cups of coffee or tea with sugar (when I say sugar, I mean any of the sweeteners we suggest such as honey and maple syrup). So, it's just about getting real with yourself and thinking about how much that sugar might be adding up over the day. Is there anywhere you could cut back? I'm not suggesting you eliminate sugar altogether but just be mindful of how much you are having in total.

7.   Are You Switching Up Your Proteins?

Meat, especially red meat, can take the body a long time to digest. Not a reason not to eat it but have a look at how much meat you are eating and try switching up your proteins to include some fish and plant-based proteins, especially at dinner.

LET'S TALK ABOUT PRE-PACKAGED AND PROCESSED FOODS

Eating pre-packaged and processed food on occasion is nothing to worry about and can be a great convenience when needed. But just like I mentioned in regards to meat and sugar, how much is it adding up? Are you eating packaged food every day...every meal? Is there anywhere you can cut back if you feel you might be using processed foods too often?

Not all processed foods are created equal. Minimally processed foods are totally fine on plan. Things like canned beans, tuna, salad mixes in a bag, frozen vegetables etc. But when it comes to frozen prepared foods, jarred sauces, condiments etc. here are some things to keep in mind when checking the ingredients.

INGREDIENT LISTS

Reading ingredient lists can seem a bit overwhelming when you first start looking. Trust me, you will become a pro! You can go down a deep dark rabbit hole when it comes to the ingredients in processed foods, so I'm just sharing some of the key things to keep in mind when shopping.

- Always avoid artificial colours, flavours or sweeteners, as well as hydrogenated oil or trans fats.

- Avoid products that contain high fructose corn syrup and watch that the ingredient list doesn't contain sugar named 3 (or more!) different ways to hide the fact that it is actually one of the top ingredients! There are over 50 different names for sugar on food labels. Some examples are: glucose, sucrose, dextrose, maltose, maltodextrin and anything ending in the word "syrup" or sugar such as "brown rice syrup" and "beet sugar".

- Always keep in mind that the first ingredient is the largest quantity ingredient and descends from there. The last ingredient being the smallest. So always look at the first 3 ingredients as they will make up the largest part of what you're eating.

- Choose the product with the least number of ingredients.

- Some of those "hard to pronounce" ingredients can be harmless and/or added in such small quantities that it's nothing to be concerned about. One example is Xanthan Gum. You might see that as an ingredient in salad dressings or sauces which is perfectly fine. It's added as a thickener and is harmless.

- When I'm not sure about an ingredient, I just Google it on my phone while I'm in the store. Or I take a pic of the list and look things up when I'm at home to educate myself.

This post is another example of how to advocate for yourself. We are all adults and have to make our own choices. I am not here to hold your hand, but I am here to provide you with the information you need to make informed choices. It's your decision, and yours alone, how hard core or relaxed you want to be about this process.

SOLE WATER

Salt is an important part of the human diet and often, when trying to be healthier, cutting back on salt seems like the right thing to do.

Salt gets a bad rap but that's because most people consume way too much of it by way of processed, convenience, and restaurant foods, which can be very high in low quality salt. "Low quality salt", like table salt, is very high in sodium, fillers, anti-caking agents and has been stripped of all its natural minerals.

While on The Program, your salt intake naturally decreases as you are eliminating or minimizing these types of foods. In fact, your desire for salt can drop altogether, leading to an even lower salt intake. That combined with increased water intake can lead to low sodium levels which we want to avoid.

WHY DO WE NEED SALT?

Salt helps balance electrolytes and helps keep us hydrated. It can aid in vascular health and a healthy nervous system. It's also important for proper muscle function and can help with muscle cramps and muscle fatigue. It can also aid in improving digestion and boosting energy. This is why it's important to maintain healthy sodium levels.

One way to make sure you are getting enough salt in your diet is to make and use Sole Water.

SOLE (PRONOUNCED SOLAY) is an elixir made up of 2 ingredients: water and natural salt. A small amount is added to your water daily.

WHY PINK HIMALAYAN SALT?

Pink Himalayan salt as well as Celtic rock salt, or other minimally processed salts, have not been stripped of any of their natural occurring minerals and don't contain unwanted additives. Regular table salt, as well as being stripped of all its minerals, is considerably higher in sodium and can also contain anti-caking agents and other additives.

HERE'S HOW TO MAKE SOLE WATER:

1. Fill a glass jar or container a ¼ of the way full with Himalayan or Celtic salt. Plastic will corrode.

2. Fill the jar with filtered water, leaving about an inch.

3. Shake it up and leave it overnight.

If using a mason jar with a metal lid, use a piece of plastic between the jar and the lid so the salt doesn't come in contact with the metal. They don't get along and the salt will corrode the metal.

If there's undissolved salt in the jar the next day that means your water is fully saturated and ready to use. You can reuse the undissolved salt to make your next batch.

HOW TO USE IT: Add one teaspoon (per day) to your morning cup of warm lemon water, a glass of water, or add it to a pitcher and sip it throughout the day. You don't need to shake it before using it. Undissolved salt means the water is fully saturated.

HOW TO STORE IT: Just leave it out on the counter!

ALTERNATIVES TO USING SOLE WATER

Add Pink Himalayan, Celtic Rock, or Sea salt to your morning warm lemon water, tea or coffee. Salt your food with the above-mentioned salts.

Purchase Trace Mineral drops to add to your water.

**PLEASE NOTE: If you have any health issues that have you watching your salt intake, please consult with a healthcare professional before using Sole water. **

LET'S TALK STRESS & SLEEP

Because managing your stress and getting enough sleep can make all the difference when it comes to getting and keeping the scale moving.

Just by following the food plan, you are helping the body manage stress because this process helps to provide an environment where the body can focus on making change and addressing issues. It also helps to calm down the body internally with the routine and structure of how everything works together.

Although the basics of The Program; the food, the water and the supplements suggested all help with both stress & sleep...there are quite a few things above and beyond that you can focus on to help with this process.

Keep in mind the goal isn't to make stress go away, it's more to recognize it, and help the body manage it, so you can capitalize on it.

TIPS FOR MANAGING STRESS:

1.   Be consistent with the basics of the program; the food, water & supplements.

2.   Practice deep breathing exercises.

3.   Get outside and commune with nature.

4.   Move your body more. Go for walks, dance, stretch, find activities you enjoy doing like sports and other leisure activities.

5.   Get better sleep:

   • The body needs deep and REM sleep to repair, rebuild and detox. You will find that following The Program will help with your overall sleep, but there are things you can do now to help make a difference when it comes to the scale.

   • Change your sleep to fall in line with the change in seasons, for example, going to sleep earlier in the winter when the sun sets earlier.

   • Take naps when you feel the need. Naps are not advised in general when trying to improve sleep patterns, but when it comes to this Process, the body is working so hard on making change so it needs all the sleep it can get.

   • Turn lights down low in the evening.

   • Use blue light glasses.

   • Stay off of screens or get off them earlier.

   • Take the calm magnesium before bed and adjust the dose as needed. It will work well with your natural melatonin production.

   • Eat as early in the evening as possible.

- Keep a journal and glass of water beside the bed.

6. Have a warm epsom salt bath before bed.

7. Keep up with health issues. Seeing a Naturopathic doctor, Chiropractor, Acupuncturist, Massage Therapist and other health care providers can be helpful.

8. Add in helpful supplements like omega 3, and add good fats to your meals along with being consistent with magnesium and any stress tonics or immune boosters you have added in.

9. Check your attitude and be self-aware of where you are at and what you are struggling with.

10. Look for things that bring you joy. Look to have fun with this process. Don't underestimate the power of having a good conversation with a friend or spending time with a loved one. Some good laughs over a glass of wine can do wonders for relieving stress.

Getting enough sleep, getting a handle on your stress and helping the body manage it, can help you to use your stress as an advantage in this process.

Stress will challenge your body and with your body working for you, it will rise to the occasion; which can lead to your body wanting to be stronger and healthier, which helps put a greater focus on fat loss.

Please take the time to head over to the Facebook Group and watch the quick video that accompanies this post.

LET'S TALK TRAVEL

How it can affect your weight loss journey and how to capitalize on it to work it to your advantage.

LET'S START WITH VACATIONS:

It's key to understand that life is stressful, too stressful for our still very primitive, working bodies. Stress can play a major role when trying to lose weight. Your body can only handle about 3 hours of stress max per day before your cortisol levels skyrocket and the next thing you know, you are blowing out your adrenals and then thyroid...leading to serious weight gain.

Members are always concerned about gaining weight when on holiday, when in fact it can do wonders for weight loss. Change in environment, less stress, abundance of good fresh foods, and some decent sleep can be exactly what the body needs to get the scale moving.

TIPS FOR TRAVEL:

- It starts at the airport...resist the urge to indulge in treats before you fly.
- Flying is super dehydrating and combined with high sugar is a recipe for carb cravings, serious bloating, and constipation once you land.
- Spend the money on healthy snacks so you are not inclined to eat the crackers and cookies or heavily salted meal they serve during the flight.
- Sometimes I buy the snacks but eat the plane food if it looks decent. I'm always happy to have the extra snacks when I land as they can come in handy.
- HYDRATE! The altitude when flying sucks the water out of you, leaving you epically dehydrated, and can have you craving carbs and sugar from the get-go...so once you land, work that water!
- Try to maintain regular eating habits as much as possible and look at any extras as just that, extra.

Generally, on vacay you are less stressed and more active in different ways, and you gotta eat right? So might as well choose foods that make you feel good.

- Don't stress if you can't follow The Plan. It's ok to have your food choices be off routine if your schedule is off from your normal weekly routine.
- Get Back on Track when you land. Start with the water and jump back on Plan. As we move forward in The Program, we will be talking more about how to help the body recover from any indulgences.
- Have fun and remember you can't do anything in a week that can't be undone with a few days Back On Track and on routine!

No one is expecting you to deprive yourself of any of the joys that come with being on vacation to be successful.

So, feel free to indulge. Just be mindful to balance it out. Try to get in fresh fruits, veggies and leafy greens when you can.

It's not unusual to lose weight while away on holiday, or to have your weight be up when you are back, only to have it drop right back down within days once you get back to following the Program or using Back On Track (which we will talk more about later). It's also not unusual for it to continue to drop to a new low afterwards.

LET'S TALK WORK FUNCTIONS AND WORK TRAVEL:

Travelling for work is not as fun but can be just as effective, as travel in general is very stimulating for the body.

- Focus on the water and keep things simple. Make the best choices you can when you can.
- Being on the road may mean making a few stops to the grocery store to pick up healthy snacks.
- Bathroom visits can be annoying, but keep in mind they are a means to an end and a key part of weight loss.
- Assess your day before it starts and plan when you can get the water in and when you need to hold off.

As we move forward, you will find it easier to plan.

TO RECAP:

Try to stay on Plan the best you can and don't stress. It's all about keeping it together when you can, balancing things out, planning ahead, and getting Back on Track when you are back.

Keep in mind that your body is not trying to or wanting to gain weight.

The key is to stay on track when you can and to be as consistent as possible. This way, you have some wiggle room for when you find yourself off or away from your daily routine.

- Consistency with supplements (if taking).
- Getting in your water when you can.
- Hitting all meals and snacks.
- Making your food choices as nutrient rich as possible.

- Being super mindful about portions, making sure you eat enough, but not too much, and allowing your body to stay focused on detox and fat loss instead of digestion.

You are working to lose weight but also to make your body healthier by increasing your metabolism, increasing your nutrient absorption, and boosting your immune system along with decreasing your insulin levels. This puts you in tune with what your body actually needs.

There is a lot to absorb here but also a super exciting time in the process so don't overthink it, have fun with it, and if you have questions make sure you let us know.

Please take time to head over to the Facebook Group and watch the quick video that accompanies this post.

WEEK 4 GUIDELINES: DOWNSIZING

THIS IS NOT ABOUT CALORIES!

Week 4 has you downsizing portions in the moment so the body feels slightly unsatisfied (after weeks of eating to satisfaction) and drops fat to adjust. You are going to keep the same routine but make your portions smaller, keeping in mind hunger levels fluctuate day to day and portions are always about what they feel like, and not what they look like.

Here we are on Week 4 of The Program...the first question I must ask is, are you still with us?

If, for whatever reason you fell off or had to take time off, I want to assure you that at any given time you pick up right where you left off. Although it is ideally followed day by day, The Program is designed in a way where you can follow at your own pace.

Any extra information you need is available in the Facebook Group and listed in descending order in the Guides section. You can also easily revisit old topics by using the Topics section.

NOW LET'S TALK DOWNSIZING

This is the point in the program that you have been working towards and waiting for.

You have spent the past 3 weeks addressing the needs of your body by giving it what it needs so it no longer feels the need to store fat.

You have worked hard to lay a strong foundation that you can now utilize to specifically get the body to focus on dropping fat!

Moving forward, this process is going to be all about the scale and your weight moving.

With that said, keep in mind we still have a long way to go and as we move forward, the formula you have been following is key and there is still very much a rhyme and a reason to each new step.

This week brings us to "DOWNSIZING"

Downsizing is my way of addressing portion sizes and decreasing the amount of insulin your body uses to break down food and ultimately, what makes you feel satisfied.

THINGS TO KEEP IN MIND:

1. **The routine of eating remains the same:**
   - Protein
   - Fruit
   - Lunch
   - Raw veg
   - Nuts/seeds
   - Dinner

2. **The kinds of foods you have been eating also stays the same.**

3. **Supplements and water intake also stay the same.**

4. **You are also still adding in and utilizing Bonus Snacks if you need them.**

5. **The only thing that we are changing is the amount of food you are eating.**
   - You do this by simply decreasing your portion sizes by a few bites less.

The goal is to get the body's attention and because you have spent the last 3 weeks eating to the point of satisfaction, even the slightest decrease in portions will be felt by the body. The key is to SLIGHTLY decrease portions, so the body feels SLIGHTLY unsatisfied.

You may feel like your portions are already small enough, but keep in mind you have been eating to the point of satisfaction for the size of body you are now. When you lose weight, you will need less food to satisfy a smaller size frame...so think of it like you are feeding a smaller size you with less weight.

In decreasing your portions by even a few bites less, the body will not be happy. It will be looking for and asking for more. When you don't give in and give your body less than what it is used to getting to feel satisfied, it will respond by dropping the extra fat it doesn't need. It drops the extra fat in order to adjust to the amount of food you are eating so it can feel satisfied again.

HERE IS HOW IT WORKS:

1. You are going to decrease portions for each meal and snack by a few bites less than you were eating to feel satisfied.

2. The body will feel unsatisfied at the end of the day for a few days, this is normal and to be expected, so you may find yourself hungry when going to bed.

3. After a few days, when you don't give the body what it needs, it will start to drop fat to adjust the amount of food you are giving it.

4. Your body will then be looking to go into detox so it can drop the extra fat.

5. Afterwards, your weight will stabilize, and the body will spend a few days working to make the changes necessary to support the fat loss.

6. You are going to downsize for Week 4, and then for Week 5 you will be back to eating to satisfaction. Then you are going to repeat the process.

**WARNING: You do not want to decrease your portions too quickly or by too much. More is not more and will NOT get you ahead. It will only slow you down.

Again, the key is to SLIGHTLY decrease portions, so the body feels SLIGHTLY unsatisfied.

****FAQS ABOUT DOWNSIZING**

1. **Do we do this every day and for every meal and snack and for how long?**

   Yes, you are keeping to the routine and sticking to the same foods you have been eating but eat a few bites less of every meal and snack. And yes, do it every day for the week and then we will bring it back to satisfaction for Week 5. Then repeat the process for Week 6.

2. **What if my breakfast is already small?**

   - Breakfast isn't necessary to eat because when you wake up you are already full of energy and any food you eat will take hours to break down before it is of any use. So, when it comes to breakfast, if you do eat it, you are breaking the fast and turning your body on, getting it to work harder from the get-go by eating higher protein.

   - You can't feel unsatisfied from food your body doesn't need so if your breakfast is already small don't worry about downsizing. If you wake up hungry and have breakfast and have room to downsize, then you should downsize.

3. **Do we still use Bonus Snacks?**

   - Yes, if you have been using Bonus Snacks, you can still use them and downsize them as well. If you have not been using them, try not to.

- PLEASE NOTE: Feeling unsatisfied is different than actually being hungry. You should NOT feel like you are starving or deprived, so don't hesitate to use the Bonus Snacks.
- BUT, before you reach for that Bonus Snack, be sure to review the HUNGER Video and keep in mind even if you are hungry, adding more food to the lineup of food your body is already digesting is not always the answer.

4. **What if I am feeling hungry at the end of the day?**

- The whole point is to feel unsatisfied, especially at the end of the day. You are decreasing the amount of insulin the body is used to getting. So, the whole point is to feel unsatisfied.
- Wrap your head around feeling unsatisfied for a few days and remind yourself this is just one phase of the program and not how it is going to be forever.
- This is just a first step in getting your body's attention, so it responds by dropping fat. You will and should be eating enough during the day even with the downsizing that you do not need to be worried about not eating enough, even if you are hungry before bed.

5. **Will I burn fat and ruin my metabolism by doing this?**

- NO. And for good measure, let me say that again, NO.
- This is why you spent the past few weeks giving your body what it needs so it no longer feels the need to store fat. This is also why the Formula and the routine is to stay the same. You will be eating every few hours so your body will be getting what it needs just not as much as it is used to.

6. **What if I don't feel that I can do this?**

- Keep in mind this is a means to an end.
- You are going to have to go through different phases to get the body to work hard and drop the weight you have gained.
- Meaning, you have to understand there is a process and you need to do what you need to do to self-correct the weight you have gained. And because you have spent the last 3 weeks giving your body what it needs and strengthening the mind-body connection, your body is going to talk to you and let you know how it feels...when it's happy and when it's not. It's important to start trusting your body.

TO RECAP:

The goal for this week is to continue to be mindful and ask yourself those 4 questions before, during, and after eating and aim to eat to feel **SLIGHTLY** unsatisfied. The goal is also to be as **consistent** as possible with the Food Plan and **maximize** your efforts day to day (refer to Maximizing Post with the 20 Questions).

I have spent a great deal of my life researching the best way to lose weight in a way that adds benefit to the body. Where you not only lose your weight, but you do so in a way that is healthy, and you can easily maintain. I would never recommend anything that would be detrimental to your health or this process, so this phase is nothing to worry about.

You are working to lose weight but also to make your body healthier by increasing your metabolism, increasing your nutrient absorption, and boosting your immune system along with decreasing your insulin levels. This puts you in tune with what your body actually needs.

There is a lot to absorb here but also a super exciting time in the process so don't overthink it, have fun with it, and if you have questions make sure you let us know.

Please take time to head over to the Facebook Group and watch the quick video that accompanies this post.

LET'S TALK SUPPORTING THE BODY IN DETOX

Throughout this Process, we have been and will be using a variety of similar techniques to help keep the body focused on detox.

"Detox" being the loose term I use to describe when the body is specifically focused on and in the process of dropping/releasing fat.

Moving forward, you will hear me talk about Supporting the Body in Detox. This refers to things you can do to help the body stay in detox for as long as possible to better capitalize on fat loss.

Outlined below are the different techniques. They are all quite similar. What sets them apart from each other is the **INTENTION** behind them, as sometimes the smallest tweak can make all the difference.

This can seem a bit confusing but is really nothing to be concerned about. This just helps to make the program a more individual process along the way. Think of it as a way to stay on top of what's happening day to day to keep things moving forward and the scale moving down.

Even if you just followed The Program as is, you will have success, so there is nothing to stress about. A lot of the time when implementing these techniques, your body is already doing what it needs to do. This just helps give you an idea of how you can step up and support the body even more.

Since we are working on DOWNSIZING, let's talk about how this would relate to Week 4.

The technique behind downsizing is to follow The Formula but to purposely eat a few bites less to leave yourself feeling unsatisfied.

The intention behind this is to get your body's attention and get it to take action:

- Consistent with supplements
- Extra water
- Hit all meals and snacks
- Purposely eating smaller portions to get the body's attention and piss it off
- Adding in bonus snacks and using heavier carbs at lunch and dinner as needed but still eating to feel unsatisfied in the moment
- Eating dinner as early as possible
- Going to bed as early as possible
- Maximizing

When in DETOX (scale moving), the focus then becomes:

- Consistent with supplements
- Extra water

- Hit all meals and snacks
- Eat even if you are not hungry, eat a token amount to stimulate the digestive system and keep things moving
- Keep portions on the smaller side to allow the body to stay focused on detox
- Lighter on the carbs and heavier on the leafy greens at lunch and dinner
- Choose easier to digest protein like fish as opposed to red meat.
- Eat as early as possible
- Go to bed earlier to help improve quality of sleep
- Move your body but keep it light, think walks after dinner. Nothing too heavy that will cause damage and sidetrack the body into focusing on repairing and rebuilding instead of detoxing.

When the scale starts to move, the intention here is to keep the body focused on detox for as long as possible to capitalize on fat loss.

1.   When your MENSTRUAL CYCLE hits:

This is a great opportunity for you to capitalize on the body's natural detox process. Your period each month is a time where the body looks to reset, to balance hormones and to get rid of any fat it doesn't need. The goal is to:

- Be consistent with supplements (Increase the calm mag)
- Drink extra water
- Hit all meals and snacks
- Keep portions on the smaller side to allow the body to stay focused on the task at hand
- Go lighter on the carbs and heavier on the leafy greens at lunch and dinner for increased roughage to help keep moving things in and out
- Eat dinner as early as possible
- Go to bed earlier to help the body get extra rest

The intention here is to help the body stay focused on the task at hand and capitalize on the natural detox process.

2.   When you are SICK:

Most people associate being sick with weight loss, when in fact with This Process, it's normal for your weight to go up (not real gain). Sickness always brings a natural detox, so there is no need to force the Formula when the body is already focused on the elimination process.

When fighting a cold or flu or any virus, the body will retain water and keep you low energy while trying to get the virus out. It will also retain and require a lot of water, which leads to the scale being up.

Also, when sick, your body won't be interested in eating, so it's normal to not be hungry.

The intention here is to help your body recover as quickly as possible and to give it what it needs so you can capitalize on the natural detox process that comes with sickness:

- Be consistent with supplements

- Add in immune support, if needed

- Add in extra water

- Be in the moment with meals and snacks, if not hungry, skip

- Keep portions on the smaller side to allow the body to stay focused on the task at hand, which is getting the virus out

- Avoid heavier carbs and go for easy to digest foods like soup to help keep energy up but not divert resources from healing

- Go to bed earlier and take naps to help the body get the rest it needs to heal

Once your appetite comes back, you can get back on track and then resume The Program. Typically, weight will drop back down and keep dropping once you start to feel better.

As you can see, the Process is similar with each situation but the intention is different. For example, when it comes to portions:

- When **Downsizing**, you are mindful of portions and keep them on the lighter side to piss the body off and get it to take action

- When on your **Menstrual cycle**, you are mindful of portions and keep them on the lighter side to help the body stay focused on the task at hand

- With any kind of **Sickness** or event that affects your appetite, you are mindful of portions and keep them on the lighter side to help the body stay focused on healing

- **Detox** in general…Once the scale is moving, you are mindful of portions and keep them on the lighter side to help the body stay focused on detox

Keep it simple, check in on where your body is at and what it is focused on, and be sure to use each technique as needed.

Don't overthink it, show up day to day and assess where you are at and what your body needs in the moment to help keep things moving.

Please take time to head over to the Facebook Group and watch the quick video that accompanies this post.

LET'S TALK INSULIN

You have heard me talk over and over about insulin in the past few weeks.

Without getting too technical, after you eat food and your digestive system breaks it down into glucose, insulin allows the body to use glucose for energy and balance blood sugar.

Insulin is a hormone made in the pancreas that regulates many metabolic processes that provide your cells with the energy they need. Understanding insulin, what insulin does, and how it affects the body, is not only important to your overall health, it's key when it comes to weight loss.

When we talk about balancing hormones on the plan, we are also talking about insulin. And when it comes to The Program, the goal is to decrease the amount of insulin your body is used to using.

**When people say they are addicted to sugar, it's not actually sugar they are addicted to. In reality they are addicted to the amount of insulin that is needed to break down sugar. **

Larger amounts of insulin are needed for larger portions of food (above and beyond what you need) & foods that are high in sugar.

By consuming foods that require less insulin to break them down and/or reducing portions so less insulin is required, you not only end up getting more nutrients from the food you eat, you can also decrease the amount of insulin your body requires overall to function properly. This will in turn lead to the body needing less insulin, which will help to decrease resistance and ultimately have you feeling more satisfied on less food.

The Rogers TV Segment I did a few years back is worth revisiting to help explain how insulin affects weight loss, plus it includes some helpful visuals

Please take time to head over to the Facebook Group and watch the quick videos that accompany this post.

LET'S TALK CELEBRATORY WEEKENDS

Because The Program covers a span of 3 months, chances are you are going to encounter these moments that are made for indulging. But with that said, they are nothing to worry about because The Program takes them into account.

We are expecting life to happen, and we are not expecting perfection, so it's more about how you want to feel after them. Meaning, how do you want to feel when it comes time to step on the scale Monday/Tuesday?

HERE ARE SOME TIPS:

1. **Take some time to set your intention before the weekend. Are you going to stay on plan, choose to indulge, or take each day as it comes?**

    There is no right or wrong answer to this, it's all about how you want to feel when it's time to get back at it.

2. **Regardless of what you plan to do, make a point of eating normally the day of any big event or in anticipation of a big/festive meal.**

    Meaning, follow the Food Plan leading up, which will help keep your digestive system stimulated so going into the meal, you digest it better, and feel less bloated after eating a bigger meal.

3. **Eating all meals and snacks leading up will prevent you from overeating.**

    Including starting your day with higher protein like eggs or full fat greek yogurt, even if you usually skip it.

4. **Starting your day higher in protein and fat and minimal carbs, for example eggs over oatmeal, will get your body working harder from the get-go and give you more sustaining energy.**

    Also, if you have carbs like cereal, oatmeal or bread, you run more of a risk of setting yourself up to crave carbs and sugar all day and if there is lots of food around, you are going to be tempted by it if you are already craving it.

5. **Stay on top of your water and try to start earlier in the day.**

    If you are on the road or out and about, make a plan and get it in when you can.

And finally, keep in mind:

At the end of the day, even if you eat your face off, you can't make a pound of fat in a day, overnight, or weekend...so all you need to do is get right back on track the next day.

Please take time to head over to the Facebook Group and watch the quick video that accompanies this post.

LET'S TALK SKIN AND WEIGHT LOSS

It's key to understand when it comes to loose skin and weight loss, it's all about how you lose it. I talk about this more extensively in the Detox Post.

When doing a traditional quick fix, burn the fat diet, you can lose weight fast. The downside is that the body takes fat from where it least needs it. This creates "pockets" or certain areas where you lose more fat than in other areas.

This is great because you can look like you have lost a lot of weight in certain areas...but it's not so great for the skin.

The key to minimizing loose skin is how you lose your weight. When you detox the fat out naturally by peeing, pooping, breathing, and sweating, you release the fat in layers. This overall gradual loss, which we use with the Livy Method, makes it much easier for the body to regenerate your skin around your new sized body frame.

HERE ARE MY TOP TIPS FOR HELPING THE SKIN DURING AND AFTER WEIGHT LOSS:

1. Dry brushing

It's like a loofah except you don't get it wet. Dry brushing is beneficial because it stimulates the nervous system, helps to increase overall circulation, but more importantly, helps to remove dead skin cells, which promotes regeneration and leaves the skin feeling invigorated.

Most experts recommend dry brushing in the morning, rather than before bed, because they believe it has energizing qualities.

Start at your feet and brush upward toward the heart. Similarly, with your arms, begin at the hands and work upward. Use firm, small strokes upward or work in a circular motion. For the stomach, work in a clockwise direction.

Dry brushing or any kind of exfoliation should be gentle on the skin, so avoid being too harsh. Ideally, dry brushing is done 1-2 times a week.

2. Collagen

Collagen is what keeps our skin from sagging, giving us that plump & youthful look. Collagen starts to decrease in the body by 1% per year after the age of 21.

Adding in a collagen supplement like the "Withinus" brand (use code **GINA15**) or the "Deep Marine Collagen" (use code **GINA20**) helps to promote the production of proteins that help structure your skin, including elastin and fibrillin.

Collagen is also found in the connective tissues of animals. Thus, foods like chicken skin, pork skin, beef, and fish are natural sources of collagen. Additionally, foods that contain gelatin, such as bone broth, also provide collagen.

Here is a list of some more food sources that either contain collagen or help promote collagen production by providing key building blocks.

- Fish
- Chicken
- Egg whites
- Citrus Fruits
- Berries
- Red and yellow vegetables
- Garlic
- White tea
- Leafy greens
- Cashews
- Tomatoes
- Bell peppers
- Beans
- Avocados
- Soy
- Also herbs high in collagen include: Chinese knotweed, horsetail, gynostemma
- Herbs that help to produce collagen include: gotukola, bala, and ashwagandha

It's hard to get what the body needs naturally so adding in a supplement is your best bet when concerned about skin issues.

Keep in mind, not all collagen supplements are created equal.

Although there are no established guidelines regarding how much collagen you should take, studies show that dosages between 2.5–15 grams of collagen peptides per day are considered safe and effective.

A better-quality product like Deep Marine or Within-Us Marine sourced collagen recommends 5 grams of powder, whereas less expensive brands might have you taking more. Something to consider when purchasing your product of choice.

You may also want to read the ingredients label, as some products may contain additional ingredients to support skin health, including silica, hyaluronic acid, or vitamin C.

Finally, be sure to opt for high quality supplements purchased from a reputable retailer. As with most things, you get what you pay for.

3. Use natural oils and creams.

Because fat stores are full of toxins from the products you use, the foods you consume and also from the environment, you want to avoid adding in more toxins by using creams on your skin that contain perfumes, dyes and synthetic ingredients.

When a cream, lotion or oil is applied to the skin, the ingredients are absorbed into the bloodstream. From there, they have a direct effect on many of the body's processes. Meaning, if the ingredients are beneficial, they'll have beneficial effects. If they are a detriment, they'll have adverse effects on the body.

Ingredients to look out for include: parabens, sulfates, petrochemicals, synthetic dyes, propylene glycol, and triclosan.

Some of my favorite natural oils to use on your body:

4. Olive oil

The antioxidants in olive oil help to soothe the skin and repair damaged cells due to excessive dryness. It can also help in preventing age related wrinkles and fine lines.

5. Grapeseed oil

Because it contains high levels of vitamin E, this oil may contribute to better skin and reducing UV damage.

6. Coconut oil

Coconut oil is a powerful antioxidant that works to eliminate free radicals that can damage your skin. In addition, coconut oil hydrates and moisturizes your skin, which prevents sagging. Coconut oil can clog pores so best to use on the body and not the face.

7. Almond oil

It's highly emollient, which means it helps to balance the absorption of moisture and water loss. Because it is also antibacterial and full of vitamin A, almond oil can be used to treat acne and some skin conditions. Its concentration of vitamin E can also help to heal sun damage, reduce the signs of aging, and fade scars.

Lastly, the things I didn't mention are all the things you are doing on Plan. Making nutrient rich food choices, adding in supplements, being hydrated, moving your body, managing your stress and getting quality sleep!

Keep in mind, right now you have your body focused on making change. A lot of the repairing of the skin happens after you have lost weight, when your body is working on stabilizing & maintaining your weight.

Just like when you cut your hand & your body repairs the skin, the same happens when you lose weight. Although it takes a while, your skin will regenerate around your new frame and anything you can do to help it along the way adds up and can make a difference.

In the coming weeks, we will be talking more extensively about skin care and skin issues with skin care experts, where you will have the opportunity to ask further questions about things like cellulite, crepey and loose skin, and skin care in general, so be sure to check into the group for that.

Please take time to head over to the Facebook Group and watch the quick video that accompanies this post.

WEEK 5 GUIDELINES: MAXIMIZING AND EATING TO SATISFACTION

Introducing MAXIMIZING, which is all the other things you can do to help the body focus on fat loss besides food, water, and any supplements.

- Duration 7 Days
- Intention to have all of your choices fall in line with your goal.
- Goal to help the body focus on fat loss and help it follow through and get the fat out.

This is an exciting time as we embark on the middle part of The Program. I hope you are enjoying the process and still as motivated as the day you started!

Over the past month, the strong foundation has been laid and the hard work is done. Now is the time to focus on the scale and maximize everything you can do to get & keep that scale moving!

FIRST THINGS FIRST:

As always, I want to remind you that even if you have fallen off plan, are behind, or have lost your motivation, it's not too late to get Back On Track.

Remember, this program takes into account off days, off weeks, holidays, and also those frustrating days where you feel like throwing in the towel.

If you are not sure how to get back at it, please let us know and we'll help you get Back On Track!

NOW, LET'S TALK WEEK 5!

This week we are taking a break from Downsizing and instead will be Maximizing and Eating to Satisfaction.

This means digging your heels in and relentlessly doing everything you can do to get the body to focus on detox, and stay in detox mode for as long as possible.

It means stepping up your game like never before, and taking everything you have learned and not just implementing it, but also building on it so you can take things to the next level.

**The goal is to take things to the NEXT LEVEL when eating to satisfaction, and maximizing to help the body focus on, and follow through on getting fat out. **

This week also helps to continue to naturally decrease your insulin sensitivity levels and get even more in tune to your portions.

Think of this week as taking everything you have learned up to this point and using it to Maximize your efforts and help the body focus on fat loss.

Week 5 is a key week because it's a jumping off point for the next downsizing week.

WHEN MAXIMIZING YOU ARE FOCUSING ON:

- Drinking your water and adjusting day to day.
- Consistency with supplements (if taking).
- Hitting all meals and snacks.
- Making your food choices as nutrient rich as possible.
- Being super mindful about portions, making sure you eat enough, but not too much, and allowing your body to stay focused on detox and fat loss instead of digestion.

**PLEASE NOTE: Eating to Satisfaction now in Week 5 is with a slightly different intention than in the first few weeks. **

For week 5, we are still asking the 4 Questions asked with mindfulness:

- Before you eat, ask yourself if you are even hungry?
- How am I feeling while eating?
- How do I feel when I'm done?
- How do I feel 10 mins later?

You asked these questions during Mindfulness & Downsizing, and now you will do the same with Satisfaction & Maximizing.

The goal is to not feel full or hungry. It's to feel like you have had JUST ENOUGH or could eat a bit more.

If you find that 10-15 minutes after eating to satisfaction you feel full, then play around with the portions. Eat what you think is enough and if you are too hungry, you can always eat more later.

We are trying to lose weight and continue to decrease insulin sensitivity levels, so portions are key.

You will have noticed after the past few weeks your portions have decreased. They will continue to be a focus, so make sure you are tuning in to them to avoid overeating.

There is a lot to focus on during this week.

THINGS TO NOTE:

EXPECT THE SCALE TO MOVE.

Remember each stage and phase is meant to get the body's attention and to get it to take action. Each week is designed to help get the body into detox and keep it there as long as possible, so your body can drop fat.

- Step 1: Get the body to focus on fat loss.
- Step 2: Create the perfect environment for the body to follow through with fat loss.
- Step 3: Support the body in detox and keep it there for as long as possible.

Obviously, there will be plateaus or stabilizing periods as they are a normal part of the process, but at this point moving forward, you should expect to see the numbers on the scale drop, even when Eating to Satisfaction and regardless of the stage and phase you are in.

Sometimes, there is a delayed reaction before the numbers show on the scale, so stick with it and keep working. Think of the end game. Getting caught up on the day-to-day numbers can sidetrack you and impact your final number.

In Week 5, you are moving from Downsizing to Eating to Satisfaction while Maximizing everything you can do to keep the body focused on detox.

This is the week where people always ask if they will lose this week or even gain weight by eating back to satisfaction.

Weight loss isn't always about eating less.

At this point, the body wants the fat gone as much as you do. The goal is to continue to support the body and give it what it needs, so it can focus on fat loss and get the fat out.

This Program is designed to help you lose weight. So, you don't need to spend any time worrying about gaining or not losing if you are following it.

This Program is successful because of my approach to weight loss. So, although it may look or feel different from the diets you have done before, that's because this isn't a diet. It's a method for helping address why the body is storing fat, so you can help it focus on fat loss and lose weight finally and forever.

SOME SIDE NOTES:

- If you have been off track, this is a great week to turn things around and get Back On Track by Eating to Satisfaction and continuing to max out everything you need to do to keep things moving.

- There is never a reason to go back and repeat steps. As long as you are attempting to make the changes you need to make each week, there is no need to repeat steps. Repeating steps can just end up confusing your body and make you feel like you're spinning your wheels.

- The program is meant to be very forward moving where one week leads into the next. The best thing you can do is to take things day by day and Maximize your efforts along the way.

MOVING FORWARD:

Lots to talk about in the coming days and some exciting weeks ahead, so continue to keep up with the Guides and check into the Facebook Group day to day.

The Check In Video moving forward is going to be more on the instructional side, so be sure not to miss it as I will be reviewing key elements of The Program day to day.

It's going to be a fun few weeks as you get closer and closer to reaching your goals! Continue to show up to Maximize each day!

Please take time to head over to the Facebook Group and watch the quick video that accompanies this post.

LET'S TALK SELF-SABOTAGE

As much as some of you want to lose weight, at this point in The Program you might start looking for a way out, a reason to give up, a reason to quit... and that's where self-sabotage can rear its ugly head. Rest assured it is perfectly normal and very common, but you will never be able to reach your weight loss goals if you don't take some time to look at this and start to pick it apart.

WHAT IS SELF-SABOTAGE?

Self-sabotage is choosing (consciously or unconsciously) to do something that undermines your success and gets in the way of you reaching your goal. The two main reasons people end up sabotaging their weight loss goals are *lack of self-esteem* and *fear*.

Lack of self-esteem leads to negative thoughts and self-talk. When you feel worthless, don't like yourself, don't believe you deserve success, or that you have what it takes to be successful, creates such negativity in your mindset. Negative self-talk can be strong and take over without you even realizing it. Before you know it you are saying to yourself or feeling like "I'll never be able to do this" "it's too hard," "I'm going to fail anyway so might as well just quit," "I'll never be able to do this," etc. ...sound familiar? This way of thinking can cause you to stop showing up every day, giving it your all, or you could end up giving up altogether.

This kind of negative chatter then feeds into your fears - the other reason you sabotage yourself.

COMMON FEARS THAT CAN LEAD TO SELF-SABOTAGING BEHAVIOURS:

Not all fears are obvious and many can be happening subconsciously. Have a look at this list and see if any of these resonate with you whether you are aware of them or not.

- **Fear of Change** - We all feel comfy and cozy in the familiar. It's hard to step outside of your comfort zone into the unknown. You may have no idea what losing weight will feel like physically or emotionally.

- **Failure and embarrassment** - Are you afraid of failing at another attempt at weight loss so might as well just give up now? It can be embarrassing to admit you have quit yet another attempt to lose weight.

- **Changing body type** - Are you afraid of what your body might look like once you have lost the weight? A body you aren't familiar with?

- **Losing Your Comfort Foods** - "What am I going to do without my comfort foods? I can't handle stress without them. I don't want to stop enjoying food!"

- **New Clothes** - "I won't even know how to shop for clothes or know what to buy! I don't have money for new clothes anyway."

- **Relationships** - "Will people be jealous of me or uncomfortable around me if they have weight to lose? Will my friends and family look at me differently or treat me differently?"

- **Fear of your abilities** - Not believing in yourself is a big one. This plays into the negative self-talk. "I can't do this" "I'm just a failure" "I just suck at this".

- **Fear of the new YOU** - Who am I without the weight? I'm afraid of becoming someone I don't know anymore. Who am I if I'm not the "fat friend" ...or sister/brother, or grandma/grandpa, or mother/father...?"

- **Looking for people to tell you what you want to hear** - Seeking out the "me too" mentality instead of listening to a good "kick in the pants".

OKAY... SO NOW WHAT? Do any of those things resonate with you? The above examples play into both categories of Fear of Failure and Fear of Success. But it's important to break those down so you can really dig into what thoughts are really holding you back. Fear of failure or success are more blanket statements that don't really get to the bottom of anything, so let's dig deeper.

You're probably also confused as to why you do such things. Especially when you're so desperate to lose weight "Why would I fear success when I've wanted to lose weight for so long?!".

Some self-sabotaging behaviours, when it comes to weight loss are obvious, like eating foods you know you shouldn't, overeating, not drinking enough water, not having your snacks etc. However, there are other behaviours that can also get in the way of reaching your goals. It's important to look at those as well.

- **Focusing on the end result instead of the journey** - Are you so focused on that goal weight that you aren't paying attention to all the other positive changes that are happening?

- **Procrastinating** - Are you avoiding doing the things you know you need to do?

- **Trying to rush results** - Are you frustrated all the time because the scale isn't moving as fast as you want it to?

- **Focusing on the scale** - Is the number on the scale going down the only thing you are thinking about? Are you stressing every time it goes up or doesn't come down as fast as you want?

- **Overthinking things and becoming overwhelmed** - Overthinking things causes unnecessary stress and ultimately makes you feel overwhelmed. Then you are tired and ready to give up… [enter stage right: negative self-talk].

- **Avoiding accountability** - Are you avoiding showing up every day and being real with yourself about what you are or are not doing?

- **Not taking responsibility and blaming others** - Are you blaming your behaviours on your family? (I'm a busy single mom), work? (I'm just too busy), on the program? (It's just not right for me, I don't like the approach).

- **Comparing yourself to everyone else** - "Everyone else is losing weight and I'm not so obviously this doesn't work for me."

- **Perfectionism** - Are you focused so much on doing everything perfectly that it's stressing you out? Do you beat yourself up every time you feel like you weren't perfect? ...leading to negative self-talk? This too causes stress and makes it easier to give up.

- **Not asking for help** - Are you avoiding asking for help, whether it's from the group or family or friends? Maybe you need extra support from your family but are afraid to ask. Maybe you don't want to ask in the group because you know you won't get the answer you want to hear.

OKAY... SO NOW WHAT?

Now, you are going to get yourself a piece of paper and a pen and go through these questions below.

1. **Ask yourself "What am I afraid of?"**

   Make a list of your own fears. Even if you are repeating some of the examples I gave above, writing them down in your own words helps it to sink in. You may also have your own fears or self-sabotaging behaviours that aren't listed above.

2. **What are my triggers?**

   What makes you turn to food other than nutritional requirements? What emotions are coming up? Angry, sad, stressed, bored, happy...can all be reasons you want to eat. Write them all down. What are you feeling, or what is happening, when you want to turn to food?

3. **How does it make you feel when you turn to food?**

   Does it make you feel better? Maybe it does, in the moment, but does it last? How does it make you feel about yourself? Write down all the negative self-talk you use when you engage in self-sabotaging behaviours. Get that negative voice out on paper so you can really take a look at it.

4. **Make a list of things you can do instead of turning to food.**

   Maybe it's taking a walk, cuddling with your pet, taking a bath, having a nice soothing tea, listening to a FB Live with Gina! Maybe it's deep breathing, meditation, yoga, listening to your favourite music and dancing it out. Whatever you can think of, that is an alternative to food. Give yourself a few options. Make a separate copy of it for easy access when you feel like you might be heading for the cookie jar.

5. **How will choosing something that's in line with your goals make you feel?**

   Maybe you don't know yet because you haven't tried, but that's okay. Write down how you think it will make you feel. After you've tried something, you can go back and add to it. Add to that how you will feel about yourself for making a different choice. How will the dialogue in your head change? No more "shit-talk" right? Huh...funny how that works!

6.   Make a list of positive self-talk/affirmations.

"You got this!" "You can face your fears head on" "It's okay to have a bad day but I can turn this around." "I don't need to be perfect" "I can and will crush this!" Pay attention to how you feel as you write these down as compared to how you felt when writing down the negative thoughts. Post this list somewhere where you can see it and read it often. Say these things to yourself every morning and every night before you go to bed.

7.   What is your WHY?

Write down all the reasons why you want to lose weight. How will your life be better once you've achieved your goal? Look back on that list anytime you are starting to feel you need some motivation.

Increasing awareness of your triggers and changing your negative self-talk is a solid first step in changing your patterns. These types of behaviours can't be changed overnight and for some are so deeply rooted that it might take more than a few lists to undo. Some of you might find that seeking out a therapist is something you need to do, and that's okay. You need to do what you need to do to stop the habit loop of self-sabotage if you want to reach your goals.

Take the time for yourself. You deserve it!

TROUBLESHOOTING: USING THE 20 QUESTIONS FROM THE MAXIMIZING POST

Troubleshooting Worksheet: Using the 20 Questions from the Maximizing Post

INSTRUCTIONS:

- Read the questions.

- Make note of the things you are doing.

- Make note of the things you can still do to help with the process.

- I suggest you give yourself an HONEST score from 1-10 on the things you are DOING, not TRYING.

- Using your score, highlight areas of opportunity that you can focus on that will amount to giving you a perfect 10.

- Once you achieve your 10, then you can rest assured that what your body needs is time.

- Check into the Facebook Group for a printable PDF of the 20 questions.

20 QUESTIONS TO ASK YOURSELF:

1. **Are you doing everything you can to create the ideal environment for your body to focus on fat loss? SCORE   /10**

    - Are you following the program 100% day in and day out? Like actually, because there is a difference between trying and doing.

    - Are you being as consistent as possible, day in and day out?

    - Have you watched these videos that break down the rhyme & reason behind the order of the meals and snacks?

        1. My Method

        2. The Food Plan

        3. Let's Talk Detox

        4. Let's Talk about the Scale

        5. Let's Talk Weight Loss

        6. Let's Talk Hunger

KEY TAKEAWAY AND TIPS:

- Checking into the Facebook Group every day and asking all the questions you need.

- Review the information over and over again until you are super clear on it.

- Making all the tweaks you need to make day to day.

- Drinking enough water for you, hitting all your meals and snacks, taking your supplements, getting enough sleep, managing your stress, and Maximizing your efforts.
- What more can you do to create the ideal environment for your body to focus on fat loss?

2. **Has your body had time to consistently focus on fat loss? SCORE** **/10**
   - Meaning has your body had days and weeks of working the plan where nothing trumps the body from focusing on fat loss? Day in and day out? Or have you had some off days and/or off weekends?
   - Be real about the time your body has had to focus on fat loss. Have you been hit or miss with following The Food Plan, sick or stressed out, or are there things you are dealing with physically or mentally that need to be taken into account?

KEY TAKEAWAY AND TIPS:

- Keep a checklist.
- Set reminders for food/water/supplements.
- Set intentions in the morning, check in mid-day, and assess your situation at night.
- What more can you do to be more consistent?

3. **Have you had the flu or a cold or any other sickness that your body is dealing with, or had to deal with and focus on? SCORE** **/10**
   - Is your body more focused on healing right now?
   - Are you taking antibiotics or meds that might mess with digestion or make you dehydrated that you need to address?
   - Are you following the Sickness Protocol?

KEY TAKEAWAY AND TIPS:

- Follow the Sickness Protocol if and when needed.
- Be patient with your body and recognize where it's at and what it needs.
- What more can you do to help your body deal with your sickness?

4. **Are you managing your stress levels? SCORE** **/10**
   - Are you meditating, deep breathing, stretching, moving your body, going for walks, taking Epsom salt baths and so on. and if so, for how long and how often?
   - Have you read the post on managing stress?

KEY TAKEAWAY AND TIPS:

- Are you really doing all you can do to help the body manage your stress? Stress can play a major role in preventing the body from focusing on fat loss. Managing your stress can go a long way in getting the scale to move.

- What more can you do to help manage your stress?

5. **Are you getting lots of deep & REM sleep? SCORE /10**

- Are you helping your body prepare for sleep by eating earlier in the evening, going to bed earlier, keeping lights low and avoiding stimulants like TV and phone, taking a relaxing bath, keeping a journal by your bed?

- Have you read the post on sleep?

KEY TAKEAWAY AND TIPS:

- Your body makes change and detoxes when you sleep. Every little bit you can do to help improve your sleep will add up and make a difference.

- Are you actually making changes? Or still staying up late? What more can you do to help improve your overall sleep?

6. **Are you drinking enough water? SCORE /10**

- Not just a set amount, but adjusting it according to the body's demands? (Not just "more than before" or "lots") Are you drinking enough?

- Are you spreading it out and sipping on it for maximum absorption & utilization?

- Are you adding in salt, sole water or trace minerals?

- Have you read all of the posts on water?

KEY TAKEAWAY AND TIPS:

- Because we utilize the body's natural detox response to get the fat out, you need to be sure you are drinking enough water for the body to be able to focus on fat loss.

- Are you Maximizing your efforts in getting in your water? Setting reminders, having a good water bottle, keeping track of your water intake through apps, elastics, or other methods.

- Get real honest here…you don't get points for drinking more than you used to, you get points for drinking as much as you actually need.

- How much daily water are you actually drinking and what else can you do to improve in this area?

7. **Are you making your food as nutrient rich as possible? SCORE /10**

- Are you adding different elements to your meals? Veg, protein, greens, healthy fats? (Not just grabbing what's convenient or easy or what you like or love. think most bang for your buck and maximum value).

- Have you read the Making Your Meals Nutrient Rich Post?

KEY TAKEAWAY AND TIPS:

- Making sure your foods are nutrient rich will ensure your body is getting the nutrients it needs so it doesn't feel the need to store fat.

- What else can you do to make your foods as nutrient rich as possible?

8. **Are you exercising? Are you moving your body? SCORE   /10**

- If so, what are you doing and how often? Are you getting your heart rate up?

- Are you making an effort to be more active?

- Are you taking the stairs, parking further away, participating and not just sitting on the sidelines?

- Are you factoring in time for the body to repair and rebuild any damage from your workouts?

- Have you read the post on exercise?

KEY TAKEAWAY AND TIPS:

- Are you being mindful to move? Is there anything else you can do to move more or make your efforts more effective

- For example, if you only have time to walk your dog 3 times/week, you can Maximize that by choosing a route that's uphill, walk with your arms above your heart to increase heart rate, perhaps carry light weights, pick up the pace, stop and do some squats along the way, etc.

9. **Are you helping the body while in detox? SCORE   /10**

- Watching portions, keeping food light, drinking lots of water, eating early at night and getting lots of sleep and maximizing everything else you can and need to do?

- Have you watched the Detox Video and read the Supporting the Body in Detox Post?

KEY TAKEAWAY AND TIPS:

- Have you made an effort to really understand and help the body Maximize when it's in detox? What else can you do to help support the body while in detox?

10. **Are you taking medications or have health issues that need to be factored in? SCORE   /10**

- You can lose weight regardless of your health issues, but they will impact your journey. So, if there are things you can do to help the body adjust to medications and help to address or heal the issue, it will help when it comes to the scale.

KEY TAKEAWAY AND TIPS:

- Be sure to work hand in hand with your doctor, pharmacist, or health practitioner when it comes to your medications.

- Get your blood work done.

- Addressing your health issues above and beyond what we are doing on The Program. For example, seeking out a hormone expert, thyroid expert, cross referencing foods that can help decrease inflammation in the body, etc.

- Have you looked into other ways you can help your body heal or deal with your health issues?

11. **Are you missing any organs? SCORE   /10**

- Are you missing any organs? Kidneys, gallbladders, thyroids, liver, have you had a hysterectomy, etc.?

- Are you helping the body compensate for missing organs by adding in the bile salts or digestive bitters if missing your gallbladder?

- Are you going the extra mile to help your body manage any deficiencies?

KEY TAKEAWAY AND TIPS

- You know your body best and what you are dealing with so you can better help support your body in all its needs, not just weight loss.

- Anything you can do to help the body better address any health issues you have will help with weight loss. What else can you do to better support any missing organs?

12. **Do you have hormone issues you need to address? Or that needs to be factored in? SCORE   /10**

- Are you seeing a specialist or adding in supplements that can help?

- Have you looked into addressing hormonal issues you may be dealing with?

KEY TAKEAWAY AND TIPS:

- Your hormones can have an impact on your weight loss journey. However, there is a lot you can do to help manage your hormones outside of what we focus on in the groups. Is there anything else you can do to help balance your hormones?

13. **Have you had your blood work done? SCORE   /10**

- Do you have any deficiencies that could be affecting your body's ability to function properly?

- Have you seen or checked in with your doctor recently?

- Have you had a physical done recently?

- Are you keeping up with appointments like your Chiropractor or Therapist?

KEY TAKEAWAY AND TIPS:

- Check into the Facebook Group for a link to a Healthline article about blood tests.
- Knowing what is going on in all areas of health in regards to your body can give you great insight into the things you can do to maximize your efforts when it comes to weight loss.

14. **Are you taking all the supplements and taking them consistently? SCORE   /10**

- They all work together and are all key in weight loss. Are you maximizing your efforts by adding them in?
- Are you consistent with taking them?
- Have you read all the posts on supplements?

KEY TAKEAWAYS AND TIPS:

- The supplements are suggested for a rhyme and a reason. They help with this program and this process.
- Have you booked a consultation with your pharmacist to discuss your supplements?
- Do you have a gameplan for when you are going to take them?
- Have you truly considered all the supplements, asked all the questions, and are you sure you have added in everything you need? Is there anything else you can do?

15. **Is your body changing? Has your body been focusing on repair and rebuild and making change? SCORE   /10**

- What changes have you seen that can't be seen on the scale and is your body changing shape and size?

KEY TAKEAWAY AND TIPS:

- Pay attention to what your body is focused on and when. The non scale victories can be just as key because your body is always working and it can't all be about weight loss.
- List some of your favourite non-scale victories here

16. **Are you eating a lot of red meat and meat in general or are you switching between veg proteins, seafood, fish, and meat? SCORE   /10**

- Be mindful about those quality protein choices.
- Are you making an effort to maximize your food choices?
- Are you choosing the best options or are you stuck on eating what you like and love?

KEY TAKEAWAY AND TIPS:

- Although there are nutrients in meat that we benefit from, meat in general can be hard to digest. It's a great idea to be adding in a variety of protein including plant based.

- What else can you do to maximize your efforts to include a variety of different protein sources in your diet?

17. Do you have any digestive issues? SCORE　　　/10

- Have you added in the supplements to help?

- Are you maximizing your food choices to help your body better digest and process your food?

- Are you eating things you are sensitive to like dairy or gluten?

- Are you keeping a journal and taking notes on how your body is responding to your food choices?

KEY TAKEAWAY AND TIPS:

- Anything you do to help with digestion will help with weight loss. Is there anything else you can do to maximize your efforts?

18. Do you have issues with bowel movements and if so, what are you doing to address them? SCORE　　/10

- Have you added in the supplements to help and are you maximizing your food choices?

- Are you making the best choices possible?

- Are you adding leafy greens to your meals and mindful to add in fibre rich foods?

KEY TAKEAWAY AND TIPS:

- Review the Bowel Movement Post and let us know if you have any questions. Although bowel movements may be all over the place - from being loose to feeling constipated - anything you can do to help with the food moving in and out of the body will help with this process.

- What else can you do to help support the body when it comes to bowel movements?

19. Are you sabotaging yourself? SCORE　　　　/10

- Do you continue to get in your own way of reaching your goals?

- Are you making choices that take you further away, not closer to, your goals?

- Are you indulging in your frustration?

- Are you having real conversations with yourself?

KEY TAKEAWAY AND TIPS:

- Sabotage is real. Be sure to review the Self-Sabotage Post for more things you can do to help with self-sabotage.

- Get real with yourself. If you recognize you are sabotaging yourself, what else can you do to help prevent it and work through it?

20. **Do you genuinely believe you have what it takes to follow through and finish? SCORE: /10**

- Do you have faith that you can lose the weight?

- What is your WHY? What is motivating you to keep showing up and to follow through till the end?

- Do you truly see yourself still here at the end?

KEY TAKEAWAY AND TIPS:

- Having a strong "why" and a strong visual of the end game can make all the difference when it comes to following through and finishing your weight loss journey.

- What else can you do to make sure you will be a success story at the end of our 12 weeks? Do you need to reexamine your WHY?

LET'S TALK SETTING INTENTIONS

This week started the conversation with a post on self-sabotage. Sabotage can mean different things for different people. Some people sabotage out of fear of failure, some out of fear of success. And some for a variety of other reasons.

Regardless, Setting Your Intentions can do a lot for helping to keep you on track each day regardless of any subconscious attempt to self-sabotage.

Setting Your Intentions in the morning is like making a declaration that you are still working towards your goal.

A reminder to yourself that the plan is to make choices that fall in line with reaching your goal, which in turn can help to keep the goal you are working towards in the forefront of your mind.

Especially in today's world with all the extra stress everyone is dealing with in their day to day, your goal of trying to also lose weight can get lost in translation some days.

Setting Your Intention first thing in the morning, checking in on yourself mid-day, and reviewing your choices at the end of the day, can help to keep you accountable to yourself.

So even if you are continually getting in your own way, this will help you to counteract that. Visualization is also key; it works like a blueprint or a guide for your body to follow.

Visualization can be done on a small-scale, day to day by visualizing and harmonizing your daily tasks, and it can also be done on a larger scale in terms of visualizing the end game and reaching your ultimate goal.

Studies show that you don't have to actually experience something for it to feel real to your body. So, if you want to take it a step further, try to also imagine what reaching your goal will "feel" like.

Making your goal feel tangible can help reinforce the belief that you are going to reach your goal.

Please take time to head over to the Facebook Group and watch the quick video that accompanies this post.

WEEK 6 GUIDELINES: DOWNSIZE AGAIN

Repeating the Downsizing process while being even more in tune to your body's needs.

I hope you are enjoying the process and are excited about the weeks to come as we move forward towards the second half of The Program!

It is even more important to stay focused as there is a lot more to cover and a lot more weight to lose!

THIS WEEK WE ARE GOING TO DOWNSIZE AGAIN.

Now, I know some of you may be wondering how you are going to downsize if your portions are already getting pretty small. Remember, when it comes to downsizing, you are only eating a few bites less from what you were eating to feel satisfied. It's about what the portions feel like when you eat, not what they look like.

It is important to keep in mind, the downsizing phase is just one of many techniques designed to get the body's attention to take action and focus on dropping fat.

The real secret to The Program and to your success is consistency with the food, the supplements, and the water, while maximizing everything you can to keep things progressing and take things to the next level.

With downsizing, the idea is to give the body slightly less food so that it feels more inclined to get rid of any extra fat it doesn't need by downsizing and adjusting to the amount of food that is coming in. This only works because of the strong foundation you created in the first few weeks by giving the body what it needs and eating to the point of satisfaction.

With downsizing, it is essential that you continue to eat all the meals and snacks that the body has come to rely on.

With the first round of downsizing in Week 4, you were decreasing portions by a few bites for a week. This was more of a practice round for you to get a sense of how it works and test the waters when it comes to eating smaller portions.

In Week 6, you are going to take things to the next level by being mindful with the portions, Maximizing everything you can to keep the scale moving, and cracking down on and testing the body a little harder now that you understand the process.

The idea is to get your body's attention and get it to focus on detox and dropping fat when normally detox and fat loss is low on the list of the body's priorities day to day.

In getting the body's attention, you may feel unsatisfied to the point where you will notice and may need to step outside your comfort zone.

**Keep in mind the idea is to feel "slightly" unsatisfied. The goal is NOT to feel hungry like you are starving and depriving your body...it's just enough of a decrease to leave it wanting more. **

Also keep in mind that you will be dealing with fluctuating hunger levels and a variety of variables that need to be factored in at any given time.

There will be some days where the body will be naturally hungrier than other days. Where one day you might be hungry every 30 minutes, and then the next day 4 hours can go by and you won't be hungry at all. Be sure to watch the Hunger Video posted in the Facebook Group.

This is normal and to be expected. On the days you are not hungry, you still want to eat a token amount. You may find after a few bites, you will start to feel hungry, in which case, you still want to leave yourself feeling unsatisfied.

It should also be noted that, although the whole point of downsizing is to see the scale move, the drop in weight may not go hand in hand with downsizing day to day. Just because you eat less doesn't mean the scale will move right away. Depending on where your body is at, and what it is currently focused on, there can be a delayed reaction in the reflection on the scale. Therefore, it is very important that you stay as consistent as possible and relentlessly MAXIMIZE and stay on top of everything you need to keep the scale moving.

ON A FINAL NOTE: Keep in mind that how you are eating now is only a means to an end. How and what you eat will change and evolve as we move forward in the weeks to come.

A LOOK AHEAD: Other stages in the program will include eating more and more often and then eating more in tune with your body's needs based on day-to-day requirements. Eventually you will be going off this structured way of eating and working on Personalizing The Plan for your own individual needs. But for now, be as consistent as you can with The Process.

If you are unsure or need a refresher on Downsizing, be sure to review your notes from Week 4 and ask any questions you need.

This is the last week you will be purposely reducing portions as we will not be Downsizing again, so do your best to be all in!

Please take time to head over to the Facebook Group and watch the quick video that accompanies this post.

LET'S TALK SECONDARY SUPPLEMENTS

The following are suggested supplements that can help speed up the fat loss process. With that said, they are not a mandatory part of the process or make or break when it comes to reaching your goals.

If you are struggling with your weight and have yet to use or add in the basic supplements, those are what you should start with first.

This list is for those of you who may be interested in taking things to the next level when it comes to your health and wellness.

You may be wondering why I haven't mentioned these products in length before now. That is because the first part of this process is to give the body what it needs so it no longer feels the need to store fat. As we move forward, it's about helping the body focus on detox and getting the fat out.

In making that the focus, your body has been working hard to re-wire and re-work how it has come to function over the years. In order to make real foundational change, it was important to give the body the time it needed to make its own connections and figure out how to rewire and re-work things on its own.

Now that you have spent the past 5 weeks laying a strong foundation, there are supplements you can add that can help take things to the next level and in a sense, speed up the process.

By no means are these suggested supplements necessary to reach your goal. Nor do you need to rush out and buy them right away to be successful.

The health food stores are full of products that promise increased fat loss, but at the end of the day, none of them will work unless your body functions properly to begin with. If you are still here, chances are your body is now working on making you as healthy as possible so it can benefit from the added support.

Read over the information and decide if you think any of the listed supplements could be a benefit to you.

**Always remember that if you have any concerns adding in any supplements, be sure to have a conversation with your healthcare provider. **

MCT OIL

MCT oil is a medium-chain triglyceride (MCT) which I started using about 15 years ago to help natural bodybuilders and professional athletes shed excess fat fast.

Coconut oil is a great source of healthy fat containing 65% MCT's, but it is important to note that when I am referring to adding in MCT oil as a supplement, I am talking about the derivative of MCT's from coconut oil...so not coconut oil itself.

The reason why MCT oil is so great for fat loss is because it works like the old thermogenic supplements people used to take to burn fat, but without the harmful effects.

Unlike every other fat source that needs to be broken down, digested, and stored before it is of any use to the body, MCT oil is easily digested and sent directly to your liver where it has a thermogenic effect and the ability to boost your metabolism (the rate at which your body functions and burns calories).

MCT's are instantly utilized for fuel instead of being stored as fat, so it helps to calm the mind (since your brain is floating in cholesterol, it needs good fat for energy to function) but keeps the body revved up and working extra hard.

Normally, MCT is a great add-in during the cooler/winter months where the body is in hibernation mode and you are looking to get it revved up.

Look for MCT oil derived from 100% coconut oil, NOT coconut oil itself.

You can take it straight up, in oil form, add to coffee and shakes, or use as a dressing on salads.

DOSE

Use as directed, although I suggest starting with 1 teaspoon and working your way up to a tablespoon per serving...to a max of 3 servings per day.

WHEN TO TAKE

Ideally, you can use it in the morning, around 3:00/4:00 pm, and then after dinner.

Side effects can include digestive upset if you use too much too soon, so I cannot express how important it is to use less instead of more, and work your way up.

Please also make sure to continue taking your omega 3 supplements, as MCT oil is not an essential fatty acid.

ADRENAL SUPPORT

Your adrenals are two nickel sized glands, just above your kidneys. Adrenals produce and control cortisol, the stress hormone. When you are stressed, your adrenals can produce too much cortisol or not enough. Cortisol is known as the stress hormone because of the body's stress response, although it is about more than just stress. Most of the cells in your body have cortisol receptors that use it for a variety of functions including: regulating blood sugar, reducing inflammation, regulating metabolism, and memory function.

We care about cortisol because too much or not enough, signals the need to store fat in the body.

THESE ARE SIGNS YOU CAN BENEFIT FROM ADRENAL SUPPORT:

- Feeling tired; struggling to wake up in the morning
- Trouble falling asleep
- Anxiety, or feeling on edge
- Mood swings
- Depression
- Weight gain
- Autoimmune issues
- Brain fog
- Body aches
- Hair loss
- Lightheaded

These symptoms are pretty general, which is one of the challenges because there are many variables that affect how your body functions.

DOSE

Follow the directions on your product's label for dosage.

WHEN TO TAKE

Take as directed and be sure to check with your doctor.

*Be sure to check in with your doctor if you are taking any antidepressant medications

WHO WOULD BENEFIT FROM ADRENAL SUPPORT?

Anyone who's been super stressed physically or mentally. Anyone with thyroid issues. Take as directed and be sure to check with your doctor.

TURMERIC

The primary antioxidant in Turmeric the spice is curcumin, which is an anti-inflammatory. While increasing your intake of turmeric isn't a lone strategy for weight loss, it may help you address the inflammation associated with extra fat and help with metabolism.

Carrying extra fat creates low grade inflammation in the body that puts you at a higher risk of developing chronic diseases, like heart disease and type 2 diabetes.

Curcumin, which is an antioxidant in turmeric, suppresses the inflammatory messaging in many cells, including pancreatic, fat and muscle cells. This can help curb insulin resistance, high blood sugar, high cholesterol levels, and other metabolic conditions resulting from excess fat.

We care because when your body isn't fighting so much inflammation, it's easier to focus on weight loss.

Turmeric is a readily available spice, and adding it to your diet has no side effects unless you have an allergy, so it can easily be added to foods.

However, in order to get the amount of curcumin necessary to aid in weight loss you would have to use a lot of it. Therefore, if you want to experience the full effects, you need to take a supplement that contains significant amounts of curcumin.

WHAT TO LOOK FOR

Curcumin is poorly absorbed into the bloodstream, so it is better absorbed with black pepper. Black pepper contains piperine, which is a natural substance that enhances the absorption of curcumin by as much as 2,000%.

The best curcumin supplements contain piperine, which substantially increases the absorption and therefore effectiveness.

DOSE

Follow the directions on your product's label for dosage.

WHEN TO TAKE

Follow the directions on your product's label.

**NOTE: Turmeric, especially taken as a supplement, can interact with certain medications, so always consult your doctor when considering adding it to your diet. Turmeric can increase your risk of bleeding if you're on blood thinners, interfere with the action of drugs that reduce stomach acid and increase the risk of low blood sugar when taken with certain diabetes drugs. Turmeric is also contraindicated if you have gallstones or obstruction of the bile passages. **

TRACE MINERALS

Most of us are familiar with the vitamins we need and know how essential they are to our health and wellness. But even with taking a supplement, or choosing nutrient rich food, many people are not getting in enough trace minerals. Even though trace minerals are only required in small amounts, they are indeed essential. Not only for good health, but also weight loss.

There are two classes of minerals:

1. Major
2. Trace

Major minerals include: calcium, potassium, chloride, phosphorus, magnesium, sodium, and selenium. Trace minerals include chromium, germanium, manganese, rubidium, vanadium, cobalt, iron, molybdenum, zinc, copper, lithium, nickel, and silica.

Minerals are needed for important metabolic functions in the body and mineral deficiencies are involved in metabolic disorders that cause diseases including hypertension, headaches, depression, heart disease, insulin resistance, and obesity.

An important part of a successful correction of the metabolism to achieve weight loss is addressing the mineral deficiency and replacing them in the correct way. Most of the over the counter multivitamins do not have the required amounts of minerals, especially the trace minerals.

Because on the program you are drinking lots of water, adding in trace minerals can also help prevent low sodium levels caused from drinking too fast, drinking too much in a short period of time, and sweating.

DOSE

Follow recommendations on your product's label.

WHEN TO TAKE

Add to your water following directions on your product's label.

COQ10

The primary role of CoQ10 is as an antioxidant. Your diet consists of antioxidants from a wide variety of sources, including fruits and vegetables.

The main source of dietary CoQ10 is from fatty fish such as mackerel, along with whole-grain foods. Your body also requires CoQ10 to produce energy from the carbohydrates and fat you eat in your diet.

CoQ10 assists in the production of energy by the cells. A deficiency can contribute to lower energy levels and a slower metabolism. Many people believe that CoQ10 production decreases with age, which can help explain one of the reasons why it can be harder to lose weight as you get older.

The CoQ10 can enhance healthy weight loss because it helps to support increased metabolic function. In addition, it can work to decrease body fat while boosting energy levels by maximizing your body's ability to convert food to fuel.

It's also great for the skin. Lack of CoQ10 results in decreased production of collagen and elastin. Collagen is important because it makes your skin firm, while elastin gives your skin flexibility. The loss of collagen and elastin causes your skin to wrinkle and sag.

DOSE

90–200 mg of CoQ10 per day is recommended, though some conditions may require higher doses of 300–600 mg. It is a relatively well tolerated and safe supplement.

WHEN TO TAKE

CoQ10 is fat soluble, so it should be taken with a meal containing fat so your body can absorb it. Also, taking CoQ10 at night may help with the body's ability to use and absorb it.

Take as directed and for more information, check in with your pharmacist/doctor.

*__NOTE: Check with your doctor if you are on blood thinning or blood pressure medications.__ **

B COMPLEX

Vitamin B complex is a group of water-soluble vitamins, which play a very important role in maintaining the growth and the metabolism of cells in the body.

When it comes to weight loss, B12 is among the MOST IMPORTANT because it helps the body convert fats and proteins into energy. B12 is mainly found in red meat, chicken, fish, dairy and eggs.

A B Complex can help the body maintain sufficient levels of a variety of B vitamins so that it can efficiently burn carbohydrates, fats, and proteins and help the body maintain energy, stamina, and control appetite.

B-vitamins are water-soluble, meaning they are not stored in the body. Though they don't stick around long, B-vitamins are vital for supporting a variety of bodily functions. Most people get the right amount of B-vitamins through diet, but others may need to supplement these important vitamins through pills or shots.

Each B-vitamin supports different bodily functions, so your doctor will be able to pinpoint the supplements you need and help you decide between B12 vs. B complex.

Typically, it is B1, B6 & B12 that is the issue.

- B1, known as thiamine, helps convert nutrients into energy, making it essential to your metabolic system. It strengthens the immune system and supports nerve function. Naturally found in pork, sunflower seeds and wheat germ.

- B2 (riboflavin): Riboflavin works with thiamine to convert food to energy, while also serving as an antioxidant. Naturally found in organ meats, beef, and mushrooms.

- B3 (niacin): Niacin helps your cells communicate and plays a role in metabolism and DNA production. Naturally found in chicken, tuna, and lentils.

- B5 (pantothenic acid): Converts food to energy, supports hormone and cholesterol production. Naturally found in liver, fish, yogurt, and avocado.

- B6 (pyridoxine): Facilitates energy production, regulates hormone activity, blood glucose levels, hemoglobin production and aids in the creation of neurotransmitters. Found naturally in chickpeas, salmon, and potatoes.

- B7 (biotin): Biotin specifically helps metabolize carbohydrates and fats. Can be found naturally in yeast, eggs, salmon, cheese, and liver.

- B9 (folate): Folate metabolizes amino acids, assists in the formation of blood cells, and helps your cells develop and divide properly. Found naturally in leafy greens, liver, and beans.
- B12 (cobalamin): Involved in neurological function, DNA production, and red blood cell development. Found naturally in animal sources like meat, eggs, seafood, and dairy.

DOSE

Range varies depending on the B vitamin. Follow directions on your product's label.

WHEN TO TAKE

B vitamins can boost energy, so it is best to take them earlier in your day and with a meal.

L-THEANINE

L-theanine is an amino acid found in both green and black tea leaves. It is also found in mushrooms, available in pill or tablet form.

It is thought to work by decreasing brain chemicals that contribute to stress and anxiety while increasing brain chemicals that encourage a sense of calm. L-theanine elevates levels of GABA, as well as serotonin and dopamine. These chemicals are known as neurotransmitters, and they work in the brain to regulate emotions, mood, concentration, alertness, and sleep as well as appetite, energy, and other cognitive skills. Increasing levels of these calming brain chemicals promotes relaxation and can help with sleep. Some research also suggests that L-theanine may improve the function of the body's immune system and help to improve inflammation in the intestinal system.

There are no known side effects of taking L-theanine. It's safe to take the supplement and/or drink teas that contain L-theanine.

Due to its calming effects, if you have low blood pressure, you may want to keep that in mind.

If you are using the Natural Calm "Calmful Sleep," it contains L-theanine. You can use magnesium and L-theanine together.

DOSE

Dose ranges from 100-400mg. Start with a smaller dose and work up.

WHEN TO TAKE

Follow the directions on your product's label.

As with all the suggestions I make, please be sure to check with your doctor if you have any concerns. For examples of products I recommend, please check the Facebook Group.

Please take time to head over to the Facebook Group and watch the quick video that accompanies this post.

LET'S TALK NON-SCALE VICTORIES

One of our Senior VAs, Krystyna Recoskie, put together this post to talk about the importance of non-scale victories. She has lost 35 lbs., is now in Maintenance, and continues to see her body change with new non-scale victories!

Non-scale victories (NSVs) refer to any changes that have improved your health and wellbeing but are not related to the scale. To take it one step further, it is any change that you are proud of that is positive and brings you joy in your weight loss journey. It doesn't matter how big or how small they may be, if YOU feel that something has changed for the better, that is something to be celebrated!

Throughout this program, we can become discouraged at times, especially if the scale is not moving. This is why we need to bring self-awareness and lean into the NSV's that are happening. If you only focus on the number the scale shows, you won't notice them! The outcome of your success is not only determined by the piece of metal, or glass lying on the floor. There are so many different things that improve during our journey to finally and forever, and we need to pay attention to those as well.

So why are the NSVs important? As Gina has mentioned before, "Your energy is your vibe." The energy you put into this program is going to affect your success. Your self-talk, and how you think and feel has a HUGE impact on this process and can impact your overall goal. Think of yourself as your own personal coach. If you are constantly giving yourself negative feedback, where will the motivation come from? Keeping a positive vibe and keeping your NSVs in the forefront of your mind throughout this process will help you realize all of your successes that have to be celebrated, motivate you, and is what will get you through the messy middle of weight loss. Remember, as long as you keep showing up for yourself, you WILL be successful in this program.

Here are some NSV examples, but remember, they can be different for everyone. Anything that you find that has improved when it comes to your health and wellness is a NSV that is worth celebrating!

- Body changing - the scale may not be moving, but your clothes feel looser. Sometimes the scale can be a bit behind when it comes to losing fat in layers.

- Improved and more regular bowel movements

- Better sleep

- More positive attitude

- Learning new information - so much info and guest speakers available to help improve your knowledge.

- Increased energy

- Being able and motivated to do things that you could not previously do. For example, exercising, taking the stairs instead of the elevator or cooking more meals.

- Mindful eating - This one is huge! Think about your improved relationship with food. Taking the time to enjoy it. Mindfully paying attention to your portions. Being IN TUNE with your body and understanding when to eat, when not to eat, and what to eat.

- Developing positive eating habits and associations
- Wedding rings fitting again
- Increased libido
- Improved complexion (hydrated skin!)
- Decreased inflammation
- Decreased or discontinued medications
- Improvement in blood pressure, sugar levels, etc.
- Positive changes in menstruation

When you are feeling discouraged, review your NSVs. Try writing them down and keep adding to the list as the program moves on. Keep them in a place where you can visually see them, so you are reminded daily and so they motivate you to keep pushing towards your goals.

Feed the positive vibes of your body and mind! Look at all of your NSVs and celebrate! The weight loss will come. This journey is about so much more than just losing weight - it is about overall health and wellness, and increasing your positive energy and vibe in life. You have given yourself a beautiful gift here - finally and forever weight loss. Keep showing up. Keep being kind to yourself, and keep celebrating those non-scale victories!

SCALE NOT MOVING? LET'S TALK 4 MAIN REASONS WHY YOUR WEIGHT MIGHT BE SLOWER TO MOVE.

The human body is not meant to store excess fat. Every extra pound of fat is hard on the body, so contrary to popular belief…your body is not looking to make you fat.

Weight gain is much more complicated than just the foods you are eating. If you are following the food plan, you are not going to gain weight. Just be mindful that for many reasons, the scale is going to fluctuate throughout this process.

With that said, this program and process will work for anyone who is human and has a body. I've never met anyone I couldn't help lose weight, as long as they were willing to put the time in and do the work necessary to make changes.

The reality is for some, weight loss will come easier and for others, they will have to work a little harder and dig a little deeper because they have some underlying issues their body is dealing with.

If your weight is dropping and or your body is changing and you are noticing non scale victories like better energy, sleeping better, and even pooping better, then chances are you are doing great and your body is responding well to the process.

There are always things you can do to level up your efforts so continue to be engaged in the conversation as we continue to focus on maximizing as we move forward with this process

If your weight isn't dropping and your body isn't changing and you are not noticing any non-scale victories, then chances are you have some issues you need to address.

4 MAIN REASONS WHY YOUR WEIGHT MIGHT NOT BE MOVING:

1: INFLAMMATION

Inflammation is an issue because weight gain is associated with increased inflammation in the body, which can lead to insulin resistance.

Insulin resistance is an issue when it comes to weight loss because it leads to higher blood sugar levels, as well as fatty liver, which can further contribute to insulin resistance.

It's key to note, there are different types of inflammation which can be caused by a variety of conditions, so it's best to check in with your Dr. as this is just a general overview.

CAUSES OF INFLAMMATION:

- Hormonal issues like insulin resistance, Hashimotos and high cortisol
- Digestive issues including food sensitivities or allergies

- Autoimmune diseases like arthritis, lupus, psoriasis
- Medications
- Stress
- Lifestyle & environment/exposure to chemicals and irritants.

It is worth pointing out there are also foods that can cause or contribute to inflammation.

These include:

- Sugar
- Refined carbohydrates
- Alcohol
- Processed meats
- Trans fats

These are foods we try to minimize and things we address while following the program. But if your body isn't responding in the way it should, then a visit to the Dr. to further investigate can be just what you need to get the scale moving.

2: FOOD SENSITIVITIES

When it comes to food allergies, you generally know when you have them as they tend to be pretty noticeable and, in some cases, extreme. Symptoms often involve swelling, itching and wheezing and can require immediate attention and medication.

Food sensitivity, on the other hand, is usually GI-related. They can happen when the body has a hard time digesting certain foods and can affect the weight loss process simply because they make people feel unwell.

They can also cause bloating and discomfort that may mimic weight gain, which doesn't help when it comes to staying motivated.

Food intolerance symptoms usually begin about half an hour after eating or drinking, but in some cases, you might not notice them for a few days after consuming.

Symptoms include:

- Nausea.
- Stomach pain.
- Gas, cramps or bloating.
- Vomiting.

- Heartburn.

- Diarrhea.

- Headaches.

- Irritability or nervousness.

As you progress through the program, you will become very in tune to your body's needs. Keeping a journal or using the Livy Method App to track how your body is dealing with the foods you eat can help give you insight into any food sensitivities you might have.

3: GUT DYSBIOSIS

I'm hesitant to use this word because it seems to be the new buzzword of the year, so it's key to keep in mind this is a general term used to describe when the bacteria in your digestive system becomes unbalanced.

There can be many causes and a variety of symptoms, so if you feel there is something off with your digestion, be sure to consult with your health care provider.

Causes of Dysbiosis:

- Consuming processed foods, including sugar & artificial sweeteners like sucralose, food additives, preservatives & artificial ingredients

- Chemicals like pesticides on unwashed fruit and veg

- Environmental toxins, skin care products

- Alcohol

- Any new medications added in

- Use of antibiotics that affect your microbiome

- Parasites

- Poor oral hygiene

- High levels of stress or anxiety

Some symptoms can include:

- Nausea, upset stomach

- Constipation

- Diarrhea

- Bad breath

- Trouble urinating

- Vaginal or rectal itching

- Bloating
- Extreme fatigue
- Chest pain
- Rashes
- Trouble concentrating
- Anxiety

There are tests your Dr. can perform to diagnose. And there are medications and different types of treatment including changes in lifestyle (like following the plan) that can help.

4: HORMONAL HEALTH

When people think of hormones, they tend to think of sex hormones, when in reality there are 50 different types of hormones that factors into your weight loss journey. These hormones control a number of functions in the body including; heart rate, appetite, sleep cycles, metabolism, mood, and of course sexual health to name a few.

Hormones are key to the weight loss conversation because your body storing fat and releasing it are regulated by certain hormones in the body. Hormones also influence your energy expenditure (or the number of calories your body burns on a daily basis, not that we care or talk about calories).

Hormones work like chemical messengers that can make or break your weight-loss efforts. While following the program, we leverage the benefits of certain hormones while minimizing the downside of others. For example, following a balanced diet that feeds into your satiety hormone (Leptin) and minimizing the need for as much insulin as your body is used to using, which are things you are already doing by following the Food Plan

Please note: I am NOT highlighting these 4 things to say that you can't lose weight if you are dealing with them. It's more so to highlight that if the scale isn't moving, there can be underlying issues the body needs to focus on more than others in order to help it start focusing on weight loss.

If you suspect you are dealing with any of these issues, have faith the program will help to address them and continue to maximize your efforts. But it is also worthwhile to work with your health care provider to level up in these areas, which can be a game changer when it comes to the scale.

Hope that helps, be sure to check into the Support Group for more info or if you have any questions.

WEEK 7 GUIDELINES: MAXIMIZING & FEEDING THE METABOLISM

Consistently working the Food Plan and Maximizing your efforts to help the body focus on fat loss. This week also has us introducing Feeding the Metabolism mid-week.

As we move into Week 7, we are going to move on from Downsizing, bring it back to Eating to Satisfaction and Maximizing for 3 days and then completely shift gears for the last 4 days.

DAYS 1-3 YOU ARE MAXIMIZING

Keep in mind that with Maximizing and Eating to Satisfaction, you are relentlessly doing everything you can to get the body to focus on detox and stay there as long as possible.

WHEN MAXIMIZING, YOU ARE FOCUSING ON:

- Drinking your water.

- Consistent with supplements (if taking).

- Hitting all meals and snacks.

- Making your food choices as nutrient rich as possible.

- Being super mindful about portions. Make sure you eat enough, but not too much, allowing your body to stay focused on detox and fat loss instead of digestion.

- Avoid eating too late in the evening. It will mess with sleep and the detox process.

- Managing stress levels, getting lots of rest, going to bed earlier, going for walks, deep breathing, moving the body and meditation.

- Being more active, adjusting workouts and adding in more movement by taking the stairs or parking further away.

DAYS 4-7 YOU ARE GOING TO INTRODUCE FEEDING THE METABOLISM. LET'S TALK FEEDING THE METABOLISM

Feeding the metabolism is meant to be used as another way to utilize your digestive system to help boost your metabolism by eating more often.

A higher metabolism means you are using more energy and burning more calories on a daily basis.

A body with a nice high metabolism looks to be as efficient as possible and looks at any extra stored fat as a hindrance and something it needs to get rid of.

In Feeding the Metabolism, you are going to continue to be super consistent with the supplements, the water, and the food. You will also continue to follow the Food Plan.

The Tweak is to split your meals into 2 portions, eating the second portion 30 minutes later. This will have you eating more often and keeps the digestive system working hard all day.

You can do this with one meal or all of your meals. You can also do this with your snacks.

FOR EXAMPLE: Prepare a lunch portion that looks right for you and divide it in two. Eat one portion, continuing to be mindful of how you feel. Later you will have the second half. If you aren't hungry for the second half, you know you have wiggle room to eat less with the first portion.

Keep in mind there is no hard and fast rule for this. You can split up all of your meals and snacks, some of your meals and snacks, or even just one.

The goal is to eat more often than what your body is used to. So, it can be once more a day to 5 more times a day, and that can change from day to day.

TO TAKE IT ONE STEP FURTHER: It is ideal when dividing meals to separate your protein from your carbs.

Protein is better digested on its own without the need for insulin, which is required to break down carbs. As an example, for lunch eat your protein first and then eat your veggies and greens later.

Do the same with vegetable protein. For example, with chickpeas, which are a protein and carb, there is still a benefit from separating them from the extra vegetables.

Healthy fats and greens can be eaten with either portion, or both.

PLEASE NOTE: When it comes to soups, stews, chili etc., where it's harder to separate the protein, just separate the portion into 2 servings and don't worry about separating the protein.

There is no right or wrong or specific time frame with this. You can eat as often as you can manage or just a few times more, and the number of times can be different each day.

- Keep in mind you are still working to maximize everything that you are doing.

- Continue to get the water in.

- Be consistent with all supplements as well as fine tuning and adjusting when needed.

- Getting as much sleep as you can since it is vital for the body to be able to detox and make changes.

- Adding in exercise or moving your body and being more active.

- Managing stress levels, meditating, deep breathing, adding in yoga and going for walks.

When it comes to PORTIONS, you want to be mindful of giving the body what it needs but also mindful not to match hunger levels. You are still looking to lose weight, so you will want to keep your portions in check. This is where you need to step up your mindfulness (ie. Keep asking yourself those 4 mindfulness questions when eating).

You don't want to purposely decrease portions to the point you stress your body like we did with downsizing. BUT, if you overeat the first portion, or even eat to feel satisfied, you will feel like you are overeating with the second portion. There is some tweaking to do here so it's important that you are paying attention.

You may find with eating more often, you are either not as hungry or hungrier. Both are beneficial responses from the body. At this point, your body wants your fat gone just as much as you do so it will be looking to get rid of it. All you need to do is stay on top of doing everything you can do to maximize your results.

TO RECAP:

Days 1-3 you are Eating to Satisfaction and Maximizing. Days 4-7 you will implement Feeding The Metabolism.

It is not okay to switch up the order of Eating to Satisfaction with Feeding the Metabolism. Everything is for a rhyme and a reason so if you start rearranging the order of things, you aren't following The Program as designed, and may not get the desired results.

As we move forward, it is normal for people to be working at their own pace due to various reasons. Regardless of where you are in the Process, getting Back on Track, Downsizing or Maximizing, we will be covering it all, so still be sure to watch the Daily Check In Videos and keep up with the Guides. If you have questions make sure you let us know.

We are only on Week 7, we have 6 weeks left to cover a lot of ground and lose a lot more weight, so stay strong and stay in the game!

Please take time to head over to the Facebook Group and watch the quick video that accompanies this post.

LET'S TALK FEEDING THE METABOLISM

HERE WE ARE ON WEEK 7

- Day 1-3 has you Eating to Satisfaction and Maximizing.
- Day 4-7 you are going to introduce Feeding the Metabolism.

Feeding the Metabolism is meant to be used as another way to utilize your digestive system to help maximize your metabolism by eating more often.

A higher metabolism means you are using more energy and burning more calories on a daily basis.

A body with a nice high metabolism looks to be as efficient as possible and looks at any extra stored fat as a hindrance and something it needs to get rid of.

LET'S TALK TWEAKS:

In Feeding the Metabolism, you are going to continue to be super consistent with the supplements, the water and the food.

You are also going to continue to follow the Food Plan.

The only thing that changes is you are going to split your meals up into smaller portions and eat as often as possible to keep the digestive system working hard all day.

- For example, you can split your breakfast into 2 portions, your lunch into 2 portions, and dinner into 2 portions.
- You can also split snacks into 2 portions each.

As you can see, this will have you eating a lot more often.

Keep in mind there is no hard and fast rule for this. You can split up all of your meals or some of your meals or just one of your meals, and the same rules apply with the Snacks.

- The goal is to eat more often than what you are used to eating. This can be 1 more time a day or 5 more times a day, and that can change day to day.
- To take it one step further, it is ideal when dividing meals to separate your protein from your carbs.
- Protein is better digested on its own without the need for insulin, which is required to break down carbs.

As an example, for lunch, eat your protein first and then eat your veggies a half hour or hour later.

With veg protein you can still do the same. With chickpeas for example, which are a protein and carb, there is still a benefit from separating them from the extra veg.

Healthy fats and greens can be eaten with either portion, or both.

For something like soup, where it's harder to separate the protein, just separate the portion into 2 servings.

THINGS TO KEEP IN MIND:

- There is no right or wrong or specific time frame with this.
- You do however want to wait at least 30 minutes. between portions.
- You can eat as often as you can manage or just a few times more.
- Keep in mind you are still working to Maximize everything that you are doing.
- Continue to get the water in.
- Be consistent with all supplements as well as fine tuning and adjusting when needed.
- Getting as much sleep as you can since it is vital for the body to be able to detox and make changes.
- Adding in exercise or moving your body and being more active.
- Managing stress levels, meditating, deep breathing, adding in yoga and going for walks.

When it comes to PORTIONS, you want to be mindful of giving the body what it needs, but also mindful not matching hunger levels or overeating.

You are still looking to lose weight, so you will want to keep your portions in check.

This is where you need to step up your Mindfulness. Remember to ask yourself those 4 Mindfulness questions at every meal and snack. You want to eat, but be mindful of portions. The goal is to eat just enough so when you walk away, you are feeling satisfied and not full or stuffed.

With breaking up your portions into smaller portions, keep in mind chances are your body will be getting more than enough food because you will be eating more often. With that said, you may find with eating more often, you are either not as hungry or hungrier. Both are normal and beneficial responses from the body.

TO RECAP:

- Be super mindful of portions, eat the first half and then take note of how you feel 15 mins later and be super mindful when eating the second half.

- If you find yourself not hungry for the second half, then just eat a token amount. This can be an indication that you may still be eating too much of your first portion. So, there's room to play around with that.

- Ideally, you want to wait at least 30 minutes before consuming the second portion.

At this point, your body wants your fat gone just as much as you do so it will be looking to get rid of it. All you need to do is stay on top of doing everything you can do to maximize your results.

Please take time to head over to the Facebook Group and watch the quick video that accompanies this post.

LET'S REVISIT EXERCISE

Exercise is a great compliment to the program, it's great for heart health, bone density, stress release as well as toning and shaping your changing body.

Earlier in the program we talked about how to incorporate it into the Program and tweak it so it is more conducive to fat loss. Because as great as exercise can be for your health and wellness, it's not the best weight loss tool. Which is one reason why it's not a mandatory component of the program. But given where we are at in the program with your body working hard to maximize your metabolism. It's not unusual for you to start thinking about moving more as your body gives you access to more energy.

Your metabolism is the rate at which your body functions day to day or to simplify, how much energy you use and calories you naturally burn on a daily basis. When the body feels a need to store fat, it keeps you in "reserve mode" and limits the amount of energy you can use.

Now that you're feeling more energetic let's talk about the best way to implement exercises that will fall in line with your weight loss goals:

- If you are new to exercise, I suggest you start by simply being more active.
- I know it sounds cliché, but things like taking the stairs and parking further away when getting groceries, going for walks or doing some push-ups or squats in your kitchen, can add up and have a big impact.
- If you are looking for something more intense, there are a lot of great home workout options. It's best to start slow to minimize the stress on the body and build up to it.
- Whatever you choose to do, it should be something you enjoy so you make a positive association to exercise moving forward and it becomes something you look forward to doing.
- You also want to walk away from any exercise feeling good and energized, not tired, taxed or drained.

You have to remember you are working towards getting the body to focus on detox and fat loss. If you work out too hard and you create too much damage in the body, it will have no choice but to focus on repairing and rebuilding instead of detox and fat loss.

When you lift weights, the goal is to rip and tear your muscle and create damage so the body works hard to fix the damage and repair the muscle making it stronger, which leaves you more toned. And that's great. However, that can very easily keep your body in a state of repair and rebuild instead of focusing on fat loss.

THIS BRINGS US TO THE TOPIC OF REST:

- If you are going to work out to the point of being sore, you need to make sure you are giving your body adequate time to repair and rebuild, or you will run the risk of over-training.

- Overtraining happens when the body can't catch up to the damage that's been done, leaving your body feeling weak and in a deficit. Which in turn can cause the body to feel the need to hold on to fat or store more fat for easy energy.

LET'S TALK CARDIO OR GETTING YOUR HEART RATE UP:

- When it comes to exercise and weight loss, it's all about the message you are sending to the body.

- Your physical brain that runs your body doesn't see what you are doing for exercise, it only interprets what you are doing based on your movements and heart rate.

- This is where you can use the body's natural FIGHT or FLIGHT response to maximize your results.

- Getting your heart rate up as high as you can for as long as you can, even if just for a few minutes, evokes the FIGHT or FLIGHT response in the body and immediately sends a message for the body to boost your metabolism and work to make you stronger.

The body's sole responsibility is to keep you alive so if you repeatedly evoke the fight or flight response, your body will look to make you as strong and efficient as possible.

In wanting to be as efficient as possible, your body will look to get rid of any extra fat that could be slowing you down.

This makes Cardio (exercise that gets your heart rate up) very effective for fat loss.

Cardio doesn't have to be running, it can be walking fast, skipping, swimming, dancing, lifting lighter weights with higher reps, sports activities, and anything else that helps get your heart rate up.

With cardio you are basically taking the muscle you already have in your body and using it to move your body, which will get your heart rate up without creating damage, making it a complement to the weight loss program.

WHEN IT COMES TO LIFTING WEIGHTS, THINGS CAN GET TRICKY:

- When it comes to lifting weights, you are purposely creating damage in the body so the body repairs the damage and makes the muscle stronger.

- That is great for bone density, building muscle and shaping your body, but not great for fat loss.

- That doesn't mean you can't continue to lift weights, especially if that is something you enjoy. I would, however, suggest you lift a little lighter using higher repetitions, to use the muscle you do have to help to get your heart rate up with minimal damage.

During sleep is when the body detoxes and/or makes change, it doesn't do both at the same time. So, if your body is always sore, then your body is always focusing on repairing the damage that is making you sore. Leaving very little to no time left to focus on detox.

With that said, you may think I'm not a fan of exercise or I'm suggesting you don't exercise….so let me be clear in saying, exercise is absolutely a benefit with this program.

The message I'm trying to get across is that you need to be smart about it and understand the message that is being sent to the body when you exercise and be mindful to support your body's needs and be sure to get enough rest between workouts.

HERE ARE MY EXERCISE FAVES FOR FAT LOSS:

- Walking because it's also conducive to healing and the least stressful type of exercise you can do.
- Anything outside, because it stimulates the brain and works the body while communing with nature and relieving stress.
- Dance or Boxing/Martial arts type classes that move the body in different ways other than side to side and up and down, while evoking the fight response.
- Biking or spinning is great for getting your heart rate up and evoking the flight response.
- Resistance training using your own body weight.

Let us know if you have any questions and be sure to check with your Health Care Provider before starting any new routine.

FOOD FACTS - ANTI-INFLAMMATORY FOODS

WHAT IS INFLAMMATION?

Inflammation is the body's normal reaction to injuries and infection. Short term bouts of inflammation called "acute inflammation" is just your body's way of protecting yourself and is doing its job just fine.

However, too much inflammation, and for too long, isn't a good thing. When this happens, the body thinks it's under constant attack so the immune system continues fighting back, indefinitely. Research has shown that chronic inflammation is linked to many diseases like arthritis, diabetes, heart disease, cancer and bowel diseases like Crohn's disease.

CAN CERTAIN FOODS HELP REDUCE INFLAMMATION?

A diet rich in anti-inflammatory foods isn't a magic cure when dealing with chronic inflammation. Medication and other treatments are important so be sure to be working with your healthcare practitioner. However, the combination of treatment and changes in diet can have a noticeable impact on low-grade inflammation.

FOODS THAT CAN HELP LOWER INFLAMMATION

The good news is, anti-inflammatory foods tend to be the same foods that help keep you healthy in other ways as well! So even if you don't suffer from inflammation, it's a great idea to add more of these nutrient rich foods into your diet!

- **Vegetables** - especially broccoli, Brussels sprouts, cauliflower, and bok choy (cruciferous veggies make another appearance!)
- **Leafy greens** - kale, spinach, and romaine lettuce. The darker the better!
- **Fresh fruit** - Intense colours are a sign that fruits are high in antioxidants. Look for dark blues & purples, like blackberries, plums and grapes. Bright reds, oranges and yellows like pomegranate, apples, raspberries, strawberries, papaya, mango and pineapple
- **Plant-based proteins** - bump up those beans and lentils!
- **Fatty fish** - salmon, sardines, albacore tuna, herring, lake trout, and mackerel
- **Whole grains** - oatmeal, dark rice's, barley, wheat kernels etc.
- **Foods with healthy fats** - olive oil, avocados, nuts, and seeds (especially walnuts, almonds, hemp, flax, and chia seeds)
- **Other foods/beverages high in antioxidants** - Ginger, turmeric, green tea, coffee and red wine (in moderation)

WHAT FOODS MAKE INFLAMMATION WORSE?

- Refined carbohydrates, such as white bread, pastries, and sweets
- Foods and drinks that are high in sugar, including excessive alcohol, soda and other sugary beverages
- Red meat
- Dairy
- Processed meat, such as hot dogs and sausages
- Fried foods
- Artificial food additives often found in highly processed foods and fast food
- Any foods that you may have a sensitivity to

BOTTOM LINE IS...

- Eat more plants
- Focus on antioxidants
- Consume Omega 3s
- Eat less red meat
- Cut out highly processed and sugary foods

If you are following the program, you have likely added in lots of great anti-inflammatory foods already. This is just another way to get you thinking about how you could level up your efforts. Whether you suffer from inflammation or not, adding in anti-inflammatory foods increases your health in general and can help prevent any inflammation from getting out of control.

LET'S REVISIT ALCOHOL

Please note: It is worth noting that your tolerance to alcohol can change while following the plan.

Meaning, if it used to take you 2 glasses of wine before you feel the effects, don't be surprised if after following the plan and losing weight that you are unable to consume as much as you did previously.

When your metabolism increases your body works more efficiently. When you combine that with significant weight loss your tolerance can change.

If you like to enjoy a beverage every now and then, here are some tips to help minimize the impact on your body and the scale:

WINE

- Choose red wine over white. Although both are fine, red has more antioxidants and is slightly better for you. That isn't a reason to give up your white if that's what you prefer.

ROSE & CHAMPAGNES

- A little higher in sugar so don't be surprised if you wake up with a headache but also totally fine to have.

BEER/CIDERS

- Avoid "light" or "low-cal" beer. Light beer may have less calories but turns to sugar faster. That is an issue because we are not worried about calories, we are more concerned about how it breaks down in the body and affects your insulin levels and digestive system. Darker beers like Guinness are higher in nutrient value but any of your regular, all-natural ales, lagers, pilsners etc. are totally fine.

- When it comes to Ciders the same rules apply. Be mindful of added sugars and artificial ingredients.

HARD LIQUOR

- When it comes to the hard stuff, be mindful about what you are using as a mix. Try to avoid pop/soda, including diet and flavoured juice.

- Stick with carbonated water, mixed with a splash of natural juices, tomato juice or Clamato etc. If you enjoy something like rye and coke or gin and tonic once every now and then, it's no big deal.

The issue with alcohol is more the food you eat with it. If you are following the plan this is a non-issue but sometimes you might be at a party and be mindfully indulging. Here's a couple of things to keep in mind if you are:

- Drinking alcohol slows down the metabolism & your digestive system, so you want to avoid any heavy carbs like bread and pasta and stick to more protein, fats (like cheese and nuts) and veggies.

- Keep in mind alcohol can affect weight loss in other ways. For example, interrupting your sleep, messing with estrogen levels, causing dehydration, and causing you to crave both sugar and salt the next day.

- Alcohol increases the production of galanin, a neuropeptide in the brain, which causes you to crave greasy food. Pair that with the effects of dehydration that causes you to crave sugar and you are ready to eat your face off the next day!

- Bumping up good fats like oils, nuts, seeds, and avocados, increasing your water along with having a banana, which is high in potassium, first thing the next day will help the body metabolize the alcohol and reduce the galanin.

- Drinking can also affect the good bacteria in your digestive system, so if your stomach always feels off the next day, try adding in or doubling up on your probiotic.

MY FINAL TIP:

The best thing you can do to offset negative effects of alcohol consumption is to add in that extra water of one cup per drink. Besides that, enjoy your beverages!

WEEK 8 GUIDELINES: FEEDING THE METABOLISM

Continuing to maximize your efforts and making the body work hard for food again. This also supports the body's need to be efficient and maximize your metabolism.

First, let me say congrats for making it this far in the Process. It is no small feat to continue to stay so focused on reaching your goals and to keep showing up for yourself each & every day!

It's an exciting place to be on this journey. After spending so much time addressing the body's needs and helping it stay focused on fat loss, your body is now in a place where it wants the fat gone just as much as you do.

Essentially, moving forward weight loss should get easier as your body is looking to boost your metabolism & make you as healthy as possible and you are more in tune than ever to your body's needs and know what it needs to stay focused on fat loss.

LET'S TALK WEEK 8

Week 8 is the same as week 7. We will be doing Maximizing and Eating to Satisfaction for the first **THREE** days followed by Feeding the Metabolism for **FOUR** days.

If you feel like you didn't have the chance to work Week 7 to the best of your ability, then this is your second chance. For a refresher, please review the Week 7 Post and check out the Video on Feeding the Metabolism, found in the Facebook Group.

OVERVIEW:

DAYS 1-3

- Back to satisfaction but with an emphasis on portions, eating just enough and being mindful not to match hunger levels.

DAYS 4-7

Feeding the Metabolism:

- Hitting all meals and snacks.

- Making foods nutrient rich.

- Breaking up meals and snacks into 2 portions.

- Separating protein from carbs (fats & greens can be included with protein or carbs).

- Super mindful of portions and adjusting to hunger levels day to day.

This will be the last week we will be following the basic food formula. Moving forward, we will be changing things up to adapt to the changes your body is making.

A LOOK AHEAD:

Week 9 - HIGHER PROTEIN AND FAT REVAMP.

Week 10 - REVAMP Part 2

Week 11 - PERSONALIZING THE FOOD PLAN.

Week 12 - MAINTENANCE & EATING OFF ROUTINE

Remember to focus on MAXIMIZING and doing all the other things, besides the food, water & any supplements, that you can be focusing on to help speed up the fat loss process.

We have a lot of time left to lose a lot of weight. Your focus moving forward should be following through and finishing just as strong, if not stronger than when you started. Your body is on your side, so continue to be all in to Maximize your results in the time frame we have left.

Please take time to head over to the Facebook Group and watch the quick video that accompanies this post.

LET'S TALK FAT

We talk a lot about fat in The Program but always in very general terms; like helping the body get rid of fat or focusing on fat loss. But we don't really talk about the different kinds of fat and what fat is used for.

Did you know there are actually three different types of fat cells in the body: white, brown, and beige. They can be stored as essential, subcutaneous, or visceral fat.

Each type of fat serves a different role. Some promote healthy metabolism and hormone levels, while others contribute to health issues.

LET'S TALK WHITE FAT:

White fat is what makes up most of the fat in your body and is also what makes you visibly fat.

It's made up of large, white, cells that are stored under the skin or around the organs in the belly, arms, buttocks, and thighs. These fat cells are the body's way of storing energy for later use.

White fat cells contain large lipid droplets and are involved with the body endocrine system:

- Metabolism
- Growth and development
- Emotions and mood
- Fertility and sexual function
- Sleep
- Blood pressure

White fat cells are found just beneath the skin (called subcutaneous fat). It's the fat that makes you look fat and tends to accumulate around the hips, butt, thighs and arms and is attributed to cellulite.

Contrary to popular belief, this is not the fat that is linked to health issues. That title belongs to visceral white fat.

WHAT IS VISCERAL WHITE FAT?

Visceral fat is the fat that accumulates around the belly, located in the abdominal cavity, and intertwined around your organs. It's this kind of fat that can increase your risk for a number of diseases.

Now, believe it or not, there is a third kind of white fat, this fat is called ectopic fat.

Ectopic fat refers to the fat that the body stores when it runs out of places to store it. Usually found in locations not normally associated with fat storage, like your liver (Fatty liver for example).

Ectopic fat can interfere with cellular function in the body, which, in turn, can affect organ function. Some of you may know it well as it's also associated with insulin resistance.

Although the body needs some white fat to function, too much white fat can have detrimental effects, and can put you at risk for health issues like type 2 diabetes, heart disease, high blood pressure, stroke, hormone imbalances, pregnancy complications, kidney disease, liver disease & cancer.

LET'S TALK BROWN FAT:

Brown fat is found in smaller quantities in the body than white fat. It gets its brown colour from iron and is denser than white fat and helps to regulate body temperature. This process is called thermogenesis. During this process, the brown fat also burns calories.

Brown fat tends to be stored around organs like your heart, liver, kidneys, and pancreas, as well as your shoulder blades and spinal cord.

Babies, for example, are born with a lot of brown fat to help regulate body temp (stored between shoulder blades).

This type of fat burns fatty acids to keep you warm. This is also why when following a program like The Livy Method, you may find ketones in your blood while losing weight.

This is not indicative of the body being in ketosis like people tend to believe, but more so of the body naturally burning fat as it's designed to do for purposes other than weight loss.

LET'S TALK BEIGE FAT:

Ok, so here's where things get a bit weird.

Beige fat is basically white fat that has been coerced by the body to act more like brown fat.

Beige fat (also known as brite fat), is relatively new in terms of research. It's believed that certain hormones and enzymes get released when the body is "stressed", for example when you are cold or even when you exercise, which can cause the body to convert white fat into acting more like brown fat.

These beige fat cells can do the job of white and brown fat cells. Similar to brown fat, beige cells can help burn fat rather than store it.

The question now of course would be how do we increase brown or beige fat cells in the body and decrease white fat cells?

The Program itself addresses the white fat cells so you already have that covered!

In terms of increasing brown fat cells, more and more research is being done on the effects of cooling your body temperature, as exposing your body to cold temperatures may help recruit more brown fat cells.

For example, taking a cold shower or having an ice bath. Turning the thermostat down or going outside in cold weather are other ways to cool your body and possibly create more brown fat.

Just keep in mind before you start purposely freezing your butt off, that the research on this is still fairly new!

Other methods suggested for increasing brown fat cells include eating more often (being sure to eat enough) and exercising to help increase metabolism, which of course we also cover on plan.

Now that we have talked about the different kinds of fat...Let's talk about the three different ways the body stores fat.

1.   Essential Fat:

Essential fat is necessary for a healthy, normal functioning body. This fat is found in your brain, bone marrow, nerves & membranes that protect your organs.

Essential fat plays a major role in hormone regulation, including the hormones that control fertility, vitamin & nutrient absorption, and regulating body temperature.

2.   Subcutaneous Fat:

Subcutaneous fat refers to the fat stored under the skin. It's a combination of white, brown & beige fat cells. Most of your body fat is subcutaneous.

It's the fat that you can grab & pinch. It's the fat that makes you "look" fat. Most notably, subcutaneous fat is the body's method of storing energy for later use.

3.   Visceral Fat:

Visceral fat, also known as "belly fat," is the white fat that's stored in your abdomen and around all of your major organs, such as the liver, kidneys, pancreas, intestines, and heart.

Too much visceral fat can increase your risk for health issues like diabetes, heart disease, stroke, artery and even some cancers.

LET'S TALK BENEFITS OF FAT:

Because as much as fat gets a bad rap, it does have its uses and benefits, such as:

- Regulating body temp
- Helps to balance hormones
- Key for reproductive health

- Ensures vitamin storage
- Important for brain health & neurological function
- Essential for healthy metabolism
- Helps to balance blood sugar

NOW LET'S TALK RISKS ASSOCIATED WITH FAT:

Having too much white fat, particularly white visceral fat, can be detrimental to your health & can increase your risk for the following health conditions:

- heart disease
- stroke
- coronary artery disease
- atherosclerosis
- pregnancy complications
- type 2 diabetes
- hormone imbalances
- some cancers

LASTLY, LET'S TALK WHAT HAPPENS WHEN YOU GAIN AND LOSE WEIGHT:

Contrary to popular belief, the total number of fat cells you have remains unchanged when we gain and lose weight. When you gain weight, fat cells expand and then shrink when you lose.

You cannot get rid of fat cells unless you have them surgically removed by way of liposuction for example. Key to note here, when you have liposuction and gain weight back, it will come back in the places where you still have fat cells, which can make for a very odd appearance.

Like all cells, fat cells do die off but are replaced with new ones every year. Once you become an adult (age of 20) the number of fat cells you have essentially stays the same.

Keep in mind this info doesn't really affect your weight loss journey and there is nothing that needs to be done with it. It is more of an FYI in the hopes of helping you guys have a deeper level of the complexities of fat & fat loss.

LET'S REVISIT THE SCALE

***We have talked a lot about the scale over these past few months, the ups, the downs and the plateaus. ***

When it comes to the scale the key thing to note is….it is going to fluctuate. Your weight loss journey will **NOT** be a straight line down.

When using the scale, it is more about the downward trend and understanding all the ups, downs and plateaus along the way.

THINGS TO KEEP IN MIND:

- When it comes to the scale using My Method, a drop is always a drop. When the scale moves down you can count on it being because of actual fat loss and that is your true weight.

- When the scale goes up it's not real weight gain. When following the plan weight gain is always superficial based on what you did or didn't eat or drink the day before. (Check out the Why is My Weight Up Post for more reasons your weight can be up)

- It is normal when you drop fat to have your weight go down & then have it go back up again on the scale as your body retains water before the cells have time to shrink It retains water because it is in detox mode and looking to drop even more, so be sure to stay on top of drinking your water.

- It is normal to wake up feeling like you have lost weight, only to have the scale showing the same number as the day before or in some cases it might even be up. This is usually a sign you are about to drop.

- It's normal to feel bloated and gross and have your weight be up the day before you see a drop on the scale. This is just the body retaining water preparing for a drop.

- If your weight is bouncing up and down the same few pounds, that usually means your body needs more water to get into detox.

- You are going to have plateaus. Plateaus are part of the process and happen when the body is adjusting to weight you have lost or is focused on making change.

- You need and want plateaus, they are necessary to help the body solidify the weight you have lost which will factor in to making your weight loss easier to maintain.

**** If you are looking to break a plateau refer to the troubleshooting post. ***

WHEN TO WEIGH IN:

- Weigh yourself in the morning after you go to the bathroom.

- Avoid weighing in at night as weight can fluctuate up to 10 pounds after a day of eating, which of course is not real weight gain

WHAT KIND OF SCALE DO YOU NEED?

- Nothing fancy, any scale will work

- A digital scale is ideal as you can see the small fluctuations, which can be helpful.

- I'm not a fan of scales that track water weight or fat % as I don't not believe they are accurate, however you can use them if you like.

OTHER THINGS TO KEEP IN MIND:

- It's key to understand that the body doesn't care about how much you want the scale to move. It has no concept of time or your desire to lose weight as fast as possible.

- Your body also has no concept of any number you want to reach on the scale.

LET'S TALK ABOUT GOALS:

What is a good weight for you?

- Without sounding cliché, I really do think it's when you feel comfortable in your skin. A good base line I use for clients is your lowest weight after the age of 21, that you were able to easily maintain.

- That doesn't mean if you have always carried extra weight that you can't weigh less than you ever have, because you totally can. I always say weight loss is a side effect of being healthy. A properly functioning body has no need for excess fat, so given the opportunity and the time, it will be more than happy to get rid of it.

- It is good to set a target weight as a goal, but I find most people underestimate their goals out of fear of failing. Group members are always setting new goals along the way and that's ok because it's a process.

- Because the body is not meant to store excess fat, there is no reason why you wouldn't be able to lose all of your weight.

- You also don't need to worry about losing too much weight as we are focused on helping the body get rid of fat that no longer serves a purpose in the healthiest of ways.

TO RECAP:

- As frustrating as it can be sometimes, the scale is a very helpful tool for weight loss and nothing to be feared.

- Best time to weigh yourself is first thing in the morning, ideally after going to the bathroom. Later in the day the scale will always read higher.

- Weight up does not mean you gained weight. It is normal for your weight to fluctuate whether you are losing weight or not.

- A new low on the scale is always real weight loss and is your actual weight.

- It's normal for the scale to be up and is usually a sign you are about to drop.

- It's normal to "feel like" you have lost weight but have the scale up or the same. This also can be a sign you are about to drop.

- It's also normal to feel bloated and gross and have your weight up the day before it shows a drop on scale.

- Weight loss is never a straight line down. The scale is going to go up and down whether you like it or not. It's a normal part of the process and it is natural for weight to fluctuate even after you have finished losing weight.

Now that you have had some time to experienced using the scale with this process, I hope this helps to not only explain, but also to normalize the ups, the downs and the plateaus when it comes to the scale while trying to reach your finally and forever weight loss goals

SELF-SABOTAGE PART 2

Self-sabotage **refers to behaviors or thought patterns that hold you back and prevent you from doing what you want to do and/or achieving your goals.**

At this point in The Program, self-sabotage can start to rear its ugly head, once again, and the reasons can be a bit different than earlier on in the process. Let's take a look at some of these and see if we can pinpoint some areas where you might be struggling. These are just a few examples with some suggestions on how you can start to address them. Awareness is the first step to change so let's get to it!

1. **I'm Rewarding Myself For Reaching A Milestone** - Many of us have been taught to use food as a reward so this one can be a tough one to break. But it is possible!

    Make a list of things other than food that you can reward yourself with. Here are some ideas to get you started:

    - A new book or magazine.
    - A new skin care product or something for the bath.
    - Treat yourself to a special coffee or tea at your favourite café with a book or a friend.
    - Schedule yourself some "ME" time, whatever that looks like for you.

2. **I've Lost A Good Chunk Of Weight So I Deserve A Break -** This is similar to #1 but a different excuse.

    Many people who are successful on Plan but haven't yet reached their goals think it's okay to start add- ing in the off-plan foods and start half-assing the process. This can be a slippery slope. Try to stay all in until you reach your goals and go through the maintenance period to solidify the weight you have lost. Don't put yourself into the situation where you lose a bunch of weight and then spend the next several years trying to lose that last 10 lbs.! If you need a break, take a mindful break. Allow yourself a "vacation". Make a plan, give it a timeline, and get right back in the game. Get it done and move on to your *finally and forever!*

3. **I'm Bored** - Bored with the food plan, the foods, the routine, the focus? Boredom is no joke and a very common reason why some people might give up.

    How about changing up some of the foods you are eating? Try a new fruit or vegetable you've always wondered about. Maybe find a new recipe to try. Remember that on-plan options are fun too! There are lots of great ideas and recipes to try over in the Recipe Share Pages in the Facebook Group. Or just try something new in general. A new hobby, a new exercise routine, take a class, learn something new!

4. **I Have 'Program Fatigue' -** You're starting to lose your enthusiasm or ambition to lose weight and maybe just plain tired of having to think about it! Take a moment to think back to when

you started and how pumped and excited you were! Why were you so excited? What is your "WHY"? Revisit that and make a list. Watch some of the Facebook Lives for motivation and inspiration. Even if you don't have time to watch all of them, checking in to watch part of one each day can really help. If you are just plain tired of having to think about it, try simplifying your meals and snacks as much as possible so there isn't much thinking involved. Prep some food on the weekends so you are prepared, set timers and reminders on your phone for your food, water and supplements. Make things as much of a "no-brainer" as you can.

5. **I'm Just Going To Enjoy The Break And Get Back In The Game In The Next Group -** There's still time to lose weight between now and the next Group! Think about how you will feel come the start date and you look back at all the time you could have been continuing with the process. Remember that even if the scale slows down because you indulge a bit more over the break, you will still have kept up the momentum, which is what weight loss is built on. This will put you in a much better position when starting the next Group or continuing your journey however you chose.

6. **The Scale Hasn't Moved, Or Is Moving Too Slowly So This Program Just Doesn't Work For Me** - If you give up now, what will you do next? Try another burn the fat diet, lose some weight, and then gain it all back plus more? Remember, even if you haven't lost any weight yet you are only making your body healthier and working towards it, eventually feeling comfortable letting go of the fat. There is no way around it, only through. Dig deeper to find what is causing your body to hold onto fat. Most often, it is an underlying health issue that can be addressed under the guidance of a healthcare professional.

7. **Future-tripping!** -You are worried about what lies ahead. How will I keep the weight off?" "What does life after weight loss look like?" "I don't trust that I can follow through and reach my goals." "I don't trust myself to not go back to my old eating habits".

    Peering into an imagined future and predicting the outcome is a major form of self-sabotage. Focusing on what you don't know isn't going to get you anywhere. Work on staying in the moment. Focus on what you need to do day to day. Practice gratitude for all you have accomplished and trust yourself to be able to handle whatever the future holds. Consider joining the next Group even if you have reached your goal to help you stay on track through maintenance. The extra support can be very helpful to not feel like you are on your own.

8. **Are You Too Focused On Numbers And The Scale Not Reaching The Number You Had Planned For The Timeframe?** - Your brain cares about numbers, not your body. As long as you are doing the things you need to do, your body will work at its own pace. Trust that your body is doing everything it needs to be doing to make you healthier. Make a list of all your non-scale victories for a reminder of all the other things you have accomplished. Do this every day to continually remind yourself. Try to take the focus off of the numbers and put it on how you feel.

SELF-SABOTAGE is no joke and often goes unnoticed if you don't take the time to stop and think. Sometimes all it takes is a little reminder of what tricks the brain can play on us to wake us to our senses! Take a step back and reflect on the things listed above. Make some lists, do some journaling, and get your head back in the game!

If you would like to dig deeper, be sure to go back and check out the first post on Self-Sabotage for even more insight and inspiration.

LET'S REVISIT WHY MY WEIGHT IS UP?

While following the Plan, your weight might go up for various reasons, none of which will have anything to do with actual weight gain.

**Let me be clear...if following the Plan, eating all the meals and snacks, making foods nutrient rich and eating to satisfaction (or even overeating) you are NOT going to gain weight. **

The body is not inclined to want to store fat, in fact it's quite the opposite. The body wants your fat gone as much as you do!

It's important to understand that throughout this Program, your weight is going to naturally fluctuate, no matter what you do.

REASONS YOUR WEIGHT CAN BE UP:

- Stress
- Lack of sleep
- Salty food
- Hard to digest food (like red meat, although not a reason to not eat it)
- Dehydration
- Body fighting an illness
- Body sore from a workout
- Body reacting to change in routine
- Body reacting to change in food
- Body reacting to new medication or change in medications
- Body reacting to any new supplements or change in supplements
- Deficiencies like being low in iron
- Hormones balancing
- PMS
- Your scale needing new batteries
- And the last, and most important reason, is your body is detoxing and your weight is about to drop.

**If you haven't seen it yet, take time to review the scale post and watch the video as it's important to understand what real weight loss looks like on the scale. **

If you stick around and keep showing up, you are going to be successful and lose your weight regardless of the little ups along the way. The ups are normal and to be expected.

Although we do like to have fun around here, weight loss can have its frustrating moments so we don't want anyone stressing about the scale any more than they need to...or even at all!

Hope this helps. Embrace the little ups because they always lead to the big drops!

LET'S REVISIT PROTEINS, CARBS, AND FATS

As we embark on Week 9 the Higher Protein and Fat Revamp, I thought it would be timely to revisit the protein, carbs and fats list.

Remember it's not an exhaustive list and keep in mind you don't need to worry about serving sizes or percentages. This is just to give you examples of what foods fall under each category.

SOURCES OF CARBS

(Foods that break down into energy)

- Fruit
- Vegetables
- Heavier Root Veg like potatoes, squash, cassava, plantain.
- Naturally occurring sugar found in things like beans and lentils and chickpeas...
- Oatmeal and whole grain cereal like hemp hearts and buckwheat
- Rice and grains like black rice & quinoa, barley
- Ryvita crackers and Ezekiel bread

SOURCES OF PROTEIN

(Feeds the muscles helping to repair and rebuild along with maintain and build muscle mass)

- Fish
- Meat (Any Meat)
- Eggs
- Seafood
- Beans, lentils, legumes
- Nuts and Seeds
- Incomplete protein like oatmeal, quinoa and dark rice (not to be used as main source)
- Dairy cheese, yogurt, milk products
- Tofu
- Protein Powder

SOURCES OF PLANT BASED PROTEIN

(As you can see below, there is protein found in lots of things besides animal sources)

- Broccoli 2.6g per 1 cup
- Asparagus 2.4g per 1 cup
- Peas 9g per 1 cup
- Cauliflower 2g per 1 cup
- Brussels 3g per 1 cup
- Bok choy 1g per 1 cup
- Spinach, collard greens 1g per 1 cup
- Mung bean sprouts 2.5g per 1 cup
- Beans (kidney, pinto, black beans, chick peas etc.) 7.5g per 1/2 cup
- Lentils 9g per 1/2 cup
- Quinoa 4g per 1/2 cup
- Tempeh 11g per 1/2 cup
- Tofu 7g per 1/2 cup
- Buckwheat 6g per 1 cup
- Soy beans/Edamame 10g per 1/2 cup
- Hemp seeds 10g per 3 tbsp
- Pumpkin seeds 5g per oz
- Chia 4g per 2 tbsp
- Nut butter -15g per 2 tbsp
- Hummus 7g per 2 tbsp
- Spirulina 4g per 1 tbsp

Keep in mind you DO NOT need to worry about these measurements. They are for reference only and to point out the fact that some proteins have carbs in them, some vegetables have protein in them, and that protein adds up.

As long as you are following the Plan as outlined, you are getting enough and the right mix of everything you need.

SOURCES OF FATS

(Essential for cellular function, providing alternative energy and brain fuel)

- Fish/Fish oil
- Omega 3 and or 369

- Alternative oils like olive oil, coconut oil, avocado oil, grape seed oil, flax and hemp oil

- Salad dressings with good quality oils

- Olives

- Avocado

- Nuts

- Seeds

- Hemp hearts

- Dairy...like yogurt, cheese, butter

This is not a complete list, it is just to give you an idea of the kind of foods I'm suggesting when talking about incorporating proteins, carbs and fats to your meals.

FOOD FACTS - CRUCIFEROUS VEGETABLES!

Did you know that the word "cruciferous" originates from the Latin word for "cross bearing"? That's because the flower petals resemble a cross.

Cruciferous [KROO] + [SIF] [UH] [RHUS]

Not sure what cruciferous vegetables are?

Here's a list of the most common ones:

- Arugula
- Bok choy
- Broccoli
- Brussels sprouts
- Cabbage
- Cauliflower
- Collard greens
- Kale
- Radish
- Turnips

These tasty veggies are packed with folate, vitamins C, E, and K and also loaded with fiber. Fiber helps to make these vegetables filling. So, a little goes a long way!

Did you know that cruciferous vegetables support many areas of our health, like detoxification, antioxidant protection, and control of inflammation? They help neutralize and eliminate toxins, providing more energy, improved health, and the power to aid in the reduction of some serious illnesses like cancers, autoimmunity, and neurodegenerative disorders.

Without getting too "sciencey" about it, they contain a sulfur rich substance called sulforaphane which is a powerful antioxidant. Sulforaphane is only activated when these vegetables are chopped or chewed. The action of "damaging" by chopping or chewing mixes the enzymes together with other components that produce the sulforaphane.

Sulforaphane can't be formed after cooking, so if you want to get the most out of your cruciferous veggies you can chop and "rest" your veggies for 40 minutes before cooking. This allows time for the enzymes to mix and the sulforaphane to be formed. Once it's there it won't be destroyed by cooking.

Cruciferous vegetables are super versatile! They can all be enjoyed raw or cooked, added to salads, soups, stir fry's, stews, roasted, steamed, sauteed, pureed...you name it!

Here are some ideas of how to easily incorporate more of these amazing veggies into your diet!

ARUGULA

It's zesty and peppery and can be enjoyed cooked or raw!

Perfect as a leafy green side dish simply drizzled with olive oil or your favourite dressing. Or toss it in your favourite soup or stir fry to add some extra zesty leafy greens.

Did you know that arugula is one of the easiest leafy greens to grow yourself? Just toss some seeds in a planter or your garden and watch them grow! They will continue to reproduce as you cut them so they can last all season long!

BROCCOLI AND CAULIFLOWER

These versatile veggies are delicious prepared in so many different ways! You can steam, roast, and grate into a "rice". Or why not try pureeing a combination of both together for a beautiful and tasty mashed potato substitute! Pick up some broccoli sprouts to add to salads for an even bigger boost of the powerful sulforaphane!

BRUSSELS SPROUTS

My fave way to enjoy Brussels sprouts is by roasting them. It brings out the sweetness. Grate some Parmesan cheese on top and you are good to go! You can also steam, or pan fry them. Brussels sprouts are equally delicious raw and make a great cole slaw or addition to any salad. Just slice them thinly or run them through a food processor and add your favourite coleslaw dressing!

CABBAGE, COLLARD GREENS AND KALE

All of the above are equally good cooked or raw. Cabbage is perfect for coleslaw of course but did you know it's also great cut into "steaks" brushed with olive oil and roasted in the oven? Collard greens... well you all know what to do with those (wink-wink) but they are also delicious chopped and fried with some oil and garlic for an amazing and easy leafy green side dish. Kale will not wilt for days so is perfect for make-ahead salads. Remove the tough stems, slice into ribbons and toss with your favourite dressing! Bok choy is a perfect addition to stir frys, soups and stews!

TURNIP & RADISH

Thinly sliced radish is a welcome peppery addition to any salad but did you know they are also delicious roasted? Roasting them releases the sweetness and mellows out the peppery bite. Turnips are totally underrated! They are very versatile and can be enjoyed raw or cooked. Boil or steam and mash as a potato substitute. Grate them raw into salads and sales or roast them on their own or with a mixture of your favourite roasted veggies to bring out their sweetness.

LET'S TALK SPRING/SUMMER: SEASONAL TRANSITION & TWEAKS

Springtime makes most of us feel lighter and brighter—and when it comes to weight loss, that feeling is real. As the temperature rises and the days get longer, your body is naturally wired to lighten up, and shed any extra fat it felt the need to store over the winter.

HERE'S WHY:

In the fall, as the temperature starts to drop and as the days get shorter, your body prepares for hibernation mode and you start to crave foods that warm you up and create heat when you eat them. Foods like soups and stews, hearty root veggies like potatoes and fatty meats are all of a sudden more appealing than the fresh fruits and leafy greens. Along with craving more carbs, the body has a tendency to store fat in the winter. Things like freezing temperatures, shorter days and lack of vitamin D reinforce that need and can make weight loss difficult.

In the spring, this situation reverses. Your body switches from hibernation mode to 'Woo Hoo! It's spring!" mode, and is looking to lighten up and drop its winter weight.

You'll notice you start to have more energy and crave fresh foods. And, as your metabolism increases and your body starts to give you more energy, you will want to move and be more active, which can make exercise a lot more appealing. To take advantage of this natural detox process, make sure you stay on top of your water game. Be mindful not to skip meals, be in tune to portions, eating just enough so your body can digest more efficiently and focus on dropping fat.

In spring, you will notice your body start to crave foods that have a cooling effect, like salads, fresh fruits and veggies, which makes it easier to keep it light and eat healthy.

Bumping up your fruit intake from one serving in the winter, to two or three + in the spring/summer, will make snacking a lot easier and can bump up your metabolism and increase your nutrient absorption, along with adding extra fibre to your diet. Because your body is looking to detox stored fat, increasing your fibre consumption is one way to speed up the fat loss process.

In the spring, your body is looking to detox and shed its winter weight and water plays an essential role in this process. You can be eating right and maximizing, but if you are not drinking enough or drop the ball on your water, then your body won't be able to get the fat out even if it wants to. As the temperature rises, you should find it much easier to drink water and stay hydrated, so take advantage. On those extra hot days, be sure to add fresh veg or fruit slices to your water, which will help it process slower and keep you better hydrated.

Late night snacking can be detrimental to any weight loss program, which makes it difficult to resist night time nibbling. When the sun goes down, the body is naturally wired to release melatonin, which helps your body wind down and get you ready for that deep REM sleep you need for weight loss.

Late night eating or snacking can interrupt that process, leaving you slow and sluggish the next day and reinforcing the need to store fat. Longer days tend to work better with work schedules and dinner time, giving you the advantage and allowing you to eat later without it affecting your weight loss goals. So play around with new dinner times so you are not eating too early or eating too late.

As the weather gets warmer, your body starts to give you more energy in order to bump up your metabolism. More energy makes exercising a lot easier and more appealing. And because using your energy creates more energy, exercise can very quickly become something your body craves and you look forward to!

Spring is also the perfect time to get outside. Fresh air and communing with nature can do wonders for your health and wellness by increasing oxygen and endorphin production along with decreasing stress levels and bumping up that natural vitamin D.

TO RECAP:

The best way to manage season transitions is to go with the flow. Adjust sleep and eating times to be more conducive to your body's natural time clock.

Be mindful of food choices, lighten up, choose easier to digest & cooling foods like seasonal fruits and veggies. When it comes to protein, ditch the fatty meats and go for more vegan options along with easier to digest fish.

Make sure to stay on top of your water and take advantage of your higher metabolism by moving your body more. With a few tweaks, the spring and summer season can be an ideal time to lose weight! And if you are going to be working on maintenance then even better, as with each season you will want to be eating in tune to your body's needs.

LET'S REVISIT TRAVEL

Although travelling can make it tricky to stay on plan it does have its advantages when it comes to weight loss.

LET'S START WITH VACATIONS:

It's key to understand that life is stressful, too stressful for our still very primitive, working bodies. Stress can play a major role when trying to lose weight.

Members are always concerned about gaining weight when on holiday, when in fact it can do wonders for weight loss. Change in environment, less stress, abundance of good fresh foods, and some decent sleep can be exactly what the body needs to get the scale moving.

TIPS FOR TRAVEL:

- It starts at the airport...resist the urge to indulge in treats before you fly.

- Flying is super dehydrating and combined with high sugar is a recipe for carb cravings, serious bloating, and constipation once you land.

- Spend the money on healthy snacks so you are not inclined to eat the crackers and cookies or heavily salted meal they serve during the flight.

- Sometimes I buy the snacks but eat the plane food if it looks decent. I'm always happy to have the extra snacks when I land as they can come in handy.

- **HYDRATE**! The altitude when flying sucks the water out of you, leaving you epically dehydrated, and can have you craving carbs and sugar from the get-go...so once you land, work that water!

- Try to maintain regular eating habits as much as possible and look at any extras as just that, extra.

Generally, on vacay you are less stressed and more active in different ways, and you gotta eat right? So might as well choose foods that make you feel good.

- Don't stress if you can't follow The Plan. It's ok to have your food choices be off routine if your schedule is off from your normal weekly routine.

- Get Back on Track when you land. Start with the water and jump back on Plan. As we move forward in The Program, we will be talking more about how to help the body recover from any indulgences.

- Have fun and remember you can't do anything in a week that can't be undone with a few days Back On Track and on routine!

No one is expecting you to deprive yourself of any of the joys that come with being on vacation to be successful. So, feel free to indulge. Just be mindful to balance it out. Try to get in fresh fruits, veggies and leafy greens when you can.

It's not unusual to lose weight while away on holiday, or to have your weight be up when you are back, only to have it drop right back down within days using Back On Track (Outlines in Week 10 Guidelines). It's also not unusual for it to continue to drop to a new low afterwards.

Travel is a challenge for the body, which is great when it comes to losing and maintaining your weight.

LET'S TALK WORK FUNCTIONS AND WORK TRAVEL:

Travelling for work is not as fun but can be just as effective, as travel in general is very stimulating for the body.

- Focus on the water and keep things simple. Make the best choices you can when you can.
- Being on the road may mean making a few stops to the grocery store to pick up healthy snacks.
- Bathroom visits can be annoying, but keep in mind they are a means to an end and a key part of weight loss.
- Assess your day before it starts and plan when you can get the water in and when you need to hold off.

As we move forward, you will find it easier to plan.

TO RECAP:

Try to stay on Plan the best you can and don't stress. It's all about keeping it together when you can, balancing things out, planning ahead, and getting Back on Track when you are back.

Keep in mind that your body is not trying to or wanting to gain weight.

The key is to stay on track when you can and to be as consistent as possible. This way, you have some wiggle room for when you find yourself off or away from your daily routine.

- Consistency with supplements (if taking).
- Getting in your water when you can.
- Hitting all meals and snacks.
- Making your food choices as nutrient rich as possible.
- Being super mindful about portions, making sure you eat enough, but not too much, and allowing your body to stay focused on detox and fat loss instead of digestion.

You are working to lose weight but also to make your body healthier by increasing your metabolism, increasing your nutrient absorption, and boosting your immune system along with decreasing your insulin levels. This puts you in tune with what your body actually needs.

Have you been travelling while following the program, if so. we would love for you to share your experience and any tips you might have below

WEEK 9 GUIDELINES: HIGHER PROTEIN & FAT REVAMP

This week is about feeding into your increasing metabolism and supporting the body working at a more optimal level.

WELCOME TO WEEK 9!

Off the heels of Feeding the Metabolism and making the body work extra hard for its food, we are going to scale back on the number of times you eat each day.

You will also be bumping up the protein and fat slightly, so your body gets more sustaining energy. I call this the **HIGHER PROTEIN AND FAT REVAMP.**

Now you may think higher fat and protein will force the body to burn fat and therefore reinforce the need to store fat. But that's not the case here.

So let me be clear **THIS IS NOT KETO.**

We will still be incorporating nutrient rich carbs such as vegetables and fruits.

The higher protein and fat will help give you more sustained energy while we scale back on the number of times you eat throughout the day. This will give the body easy energy which will feed into its need to easily work at a more optimal level.

You will still be following the Food Plan Formula but we will be making a few tweaks.

With where we are in The Program, your body is working hard to boost your metabolism. Decreasing the number of times you are eating each day along with increasing protein and fat will feed into your increasing metabolism, which will cause the body to decrease insulin levels even further.

Portion wise, the goal is still to just eat JUST ENOUGH, so 10-15 min later you don't feel full or stuffed.

THIS WEEK'S TWEAK:

Breakfast - still higher protein, ideally taking out any harder to digest carbs like bread, crackers, oatmeal's and go more for fish, eggs, yogurts, protein shakes, etc.

Morning Snack - can still be fruit but with added protein and fat. OR you can skip the fruit and just have protein and fat (examples below).

Lunch - protein is now the star of the show with veg and leafy greens. Eliminate any heavier carbs like potatoes, white rice, grains... except quinoa & black rice in small portions if needed.

Afternoon Snack (only one) - There will only be one afternoon snack. You can combine the veg and nuts/seeds snack or see other ideas/options below.

Dinner - Veg. is now the star of the show with protein and leafy greens. Please note the added carbs by way of the vegetables, which are now the star of the show at dinner. This will help balance out the day of eating higher protein.

Let's revisit PROTEIN & FAT sources:

PROTEIN SOURCES:

- Fish
- Meat (Any Meat)
- Eggs
- Seafood
- Beans, lentils, legumes
- Nuts and Seeds
- Dairy cheese, yogurt, milk products
- Tofu, Tempeh
- Nut butter
- Hummus
- All-natural protein powder
- …and don't forget about the protein in the vegetable carbs you are eating!

FAT SOURCES:

- Olives
- Avocado
- Nuts
- Seeds
- Hemp hearts
- Dairy...like yogurt, cheese, butter, sour cream etc.
- Olive oil, coconut oil, avocado oil, grape seed oil, flax and hemp oil
- Salad dressings made with good quality oils
- Omega 3 and 369
- Plus, any others you might think of

MEAL AND SNACK EXAMPLES/IDEAS:

**Keep in mind these are only ideas. Feel free to come up with your own. **

BREAKFAST:

- Eggs and egg whites (can add sautéed veg and/or greens)
- Yogurt with hemp hearts nuts/seeds. Can also add protein powder.
- Beans or lentils
- Veg or meat protein (can add sautéed veg)
- Higher protein cereals such as Holy Crap or Andrea's Killer Grain Cereal with added hemp hearts.
- Protein shakes (make sure to use natural protein powders). If adding fruit, keep it to a minimum and add in good fat by way of oils, avocados, nut butter, nuts, seeds, unsweetened coconut, coconut milk etc.

MORNING SNACK IDEAS:

- Fruit with nuts, seeds, nut butter, cheese or avocado
- Nuts and/or seeds on their own
- Yogurt
- Boiled egg
- Protein shake (If you didn't have it for breakfast) make sure to use natural protein powders. If adding fruit, keep it to a minimum and add in good fat by way of oils, avocados, coconut etc.

LUNCH:

- Take out any heavier carbs like potatoes, white rice, grains... except quinoa & black rice in small portions if needed, or other whole grains such as spelt, kamut, teff, amaranth, sorghum etc.

- Protein (any kind) with veg/leafy greens in any combination of soup, salad, stew, stir fry or just straight up.

AFTERNOON SNACK IDEAS:

- Raw veg with nuts and/or seeds

- Nuts, seeds, or cheese

- Yogurt, cottage cheese (if you didn't have it in the AM)

- Raw veg with natural dips, guacamole, hummus, or nut butter

- Fruit and protein (like nuts, cheese, boiled eggs)

DINNER:

- Veg, protein, leafy greens (protein should be a smaller portion and veg is now the star of the show.

It's a few simple tweaks, so try not to overthink it. Although you want to be super mindful of portions, try to avoid purposely trying to eat less. Taking out the heavier carbs will do the work for you, so make sure to eat to satisfaction (JUST ENOUGH) and still be mindful of portions.

You may find portions may be smaller or larger this week. Both are normal responses from the body and as always, hunger levels change day to day and portions are always what they feel like and not what they look like.

Please take time to head over to the Facebook Group and watch the quick video that accompanies this post.

LET'S TALK PROTEIN SHAKES

I think I have made my stance on shakes pretty clear. It's not that I'm opposed to having them, it's just when it comes to weight loss...there is a time and a place for them.

With where we are at in the Process, and with the focus more on supporting the body where it is at and feeding into its increasing metabolism...protein shakes can be an easy and convenient way for the body to get what it needs so it can better focus on fat loss.

If you are thinking of adding in a shake here are some things to keep in mind:

1.   There are a variety of protein powder options out there, find one that works best for you.

SIDE NOTE: Although shakes can be the perfect place to add in your collagen powder, collagen powder is a non-essential protein (not a food source) so it doesn't replace the need for protein powder in a shake.

2.   Check the ingredients, make sure you are buying natural protein powder (not synthetic) and avoid any artificial flavour or colour or sweeteners.

3.   Make sure to add in good fat which will balance out any carbs (fruits or veg) you add in. Examples of some good fats would be:

- Liquid Omega 3 or 369 combo
- Flax oil
- Hemp oil
- Avocado
- Coconut oil/chunks, or unsweetened milk
- MCT oil
- Nut butters
- Yogurt

4.   Be mindful about the amount of fruit ratio you are using and bonus if you make them more veg based.

5.   Be in tune to the portion size of your shake, with liquid nutrients you need less than what you would eat because the breakdown process is already done for you.

Keep in mind you do NOT need to add in protein shakes. You can get everything you need to be successful with this week's tweak without adding them in. However...if you are a fan of shakes and looking to add them in, be sure to check into the Facebook Group for some shared recipes.

Please take time to head over to the Facebook Group and watch the quick video that accompanies this post.

LET'S REVISIT NUTRIENT RICH MEALS

With where we are in the program, it's easy to fall into old habits and start choosing foods that you like and love or are easy and convenient instead of choosing foods that will maximize your efforts.

Not that this program is all about salads but if you are going to eat them, make sure you load them up with tons of nutrients, think quality over quantity.

Let's use the salad in the photo as an example, but the same idea can be applied to absolutely ANY meal and even your snacks.

LET'S BREAK IT DOWN:

- Spring Mix/Greens = leafy greens + roughage + vitamins + minerals + protein
- Variety of Vegetables = fiber + vitamins
- Avocado = healthy fat + potassium + fiber
- Feta cheese = healthy fat + protein
- Nuts and Seeds = healthy fat + protein
- Honey Mustard Dressing = healthy fat when made with quality oil.

Nutrient rich meals provide the most bang for your buck and give you longer lasting energy.

Even if you can just sneak in one or two extra things like a drizzle of olive oil, an extra veg, or a few nuts… it can make all the difference.

THINGS TO HAVE ON HAND THAT CAN QUICKLY BUMP UP YOUR MEALS:

- A variety of nuts and seeds - good fat and protein and an excellent addition to yogurt or oats
- Olives - good fat
- Pickled and marinated veg like artichoke heart, pickled beets, roasted red peppers, etc. - bump up your veggies.
- Good quality oils like extra virgin olive oil, nut oils, avocado and coconut oil. - good fats
- Quality salad dressings (store bought or homemade) - good fat
- Coconut milk - a great healthy fat addition to things like your morning oatmeal or cereal.
- Salsa - extra veg
- Guacamole - good fat
- Hummus - good fat plus protein
- Tuna, sardines, smoked oysters a quick way - to add protein to any meal.

LET'S REVISIT STRESS & SLEEP

Stress factors into the weight loss process because when you are stressed your body releases a hormone called cortisol and too much cortisol can signal weight gain.

Sleep is key to the process because when you sleep is when the body makes all the changes you want to see.

Managing your stress and getting enough sleep can make all the difference when it comes to getting and keeping the scale moving.

Just by following the food plan, you are helping the body manage stress because this process helps to provide an environment where the body can focus on making change and addressing issues.

Although the basics of The Program; the food, the water and the supplements suggested all help with both stress & sleep...there are quite a few things above and beyond that you can focus on to help with this process.

TIPS FOR MANAGING STRESS:

1. Be consistent with the basics of the program; the food, water & supplements.

2. Practice deep breathing exercises.

3. Get outside and commune with nature.

4. Move your body more. Go for walks, dance, stretch, find activities you enjoy doing like sports and other leisure activities.

5. Have a warm epsom salt bath before bed.

6. Keep up with health issues. Seeing a Naturopathic doctor, Chiropractor, Acupuncturist, Massage Therapist and other health care providers can be helpful.

7. Add in helpful supplements like omega 3, and add good fats to your meals along with being consistent with magnesium and any stress tonics or immune boosters you have added in.

8. Check your attitude and be self-aware of where you are at and what you are struggling with. Help you help yourself and prioritize your body's needs.

9. Look for things that bring you joy. Look to have fun with this process. Don't underestimate the power of having a good conversation with a friend or spending time with a loved one. Some good laughs over a glass of wine can do wonders for relieving stress.

10. Get better sleep:

The body needs deep and REM sleep to repair, rebuild and detox. You will find that following The Program will help with your overall sleep, but there are things you can do now to help make a difference when it comes to the scale.

- Change your sleep to fall in line with the change in seasons, for example, going to sleep earlier in the fall when the sun sets earlier.

- Take naps when you feel the need. Naps are not advised in general when trying to improve sleep patterns, but when it comes to this Process, the body is working so hard on making change, it needs all the sleep it can get.

- Turn lights down low in the evening.

- Use blue light glasses.

- Stay off of screens or get off them earlier.

- Add in the calm magnesium before bed and adjust the dose as needed. It will work well with your natural melatonin production.

- Eat as early in the evening as possible.

- Keep a journal and glass of water beside the bed.

Getting enough sleep, getting a handle on your stress and helping the body manage it, can help you to use your stress as an advantage in this process.

Stress will challenge your body and with your body working for you, it will rise to the occasion; which can lead to your body wanting to be stronger and healthier, which helps put a greater focus on fat loss.

Keep in mind the goal isn't to make stress go away, it's more to recognize it, and help the body manage it, so you can capitalize on it. And when it comes to sleep you may not be able to get more sleep but you can work to improve the quality of sleep you do get.

LET'S REVISIT KEEPING A JOURNAL

It's not too late to start tracking your progress.

We have talked in the past about the benefits of keeping a journal or using our app to track things like your weight to see patterns of behavior and how your body responds to this process. Also, the importance of tracking things like how you feel physically and mentally as well as the basics like your water to help make sure you are drinking enough.

But it can be even more important with where we are at in this process now to help you capitalize on the time we have left…which, by the way, is still a lot of time left to lose a lot of weight!

BENEFITS OF JOURNALING:

- A journal can be a great tool to help give you insight into how your body is responding to the process.
- It can help you pick up on patterns of behavior and responses, and give you a better idea of what weight loss looks like specifically to you.
- It can help you pick up on any food sensitivities, especially if you have digestive issues. It can help you track bowel movements if you struggle in that department.
- It can help you track your body's response to the supplements you have been taking and/or anything new you are adding in or taking out.
- It can also help to track your mood and can be beneficial in helping you show up for yourself every day, by taking time to think about how you are managing your emotions and how you are feeling day to day.

THINGS TO TRACK:

- Weight in the morning
- How you are feeling physically and mentally
- Food
- Water
- Extras (added food and drink on or not on plan)
- Bowel movements if they are an issue
- Notable responses from food
- Digestive upset
- Sleep
- Medications

- Supplements

- Notable wins not food related (NSV)

- Energy day to day

- Changes taking place that aren't scale related

You can use good old pen and paper, your computer, or an app. Whatever works best for you!

We are at the point in this process where keeping a journal can be a very helpful tool to problem solve and make the most of your effort in conjunction with the info being posted in the group.

The more tools the better!

FOOD FACTS - BEANS & LENTILS

How many of you are familiar with these 2 rhymes?

"Beans, beans, they're good for your heart

The more you eat, the more you fart,

The more you fart the better you feel

So, eat some beans with every meal!"

"Beans, beans the musical fruit, the more you eat, the less you toot!"

My grandfather used to recite both of these to me when I was a kid anytime I was eating beans (usually beans and wieners!). It always made me giggle. But did you notice how the 2 rhymes say opposite things about gassiness?

SO WHICH ONE IS IT?

Well...sort of both. Beans and lentils *can* cause an increase in gassiness after eating. This is because of a complex sugar called raffinose, which the body can have trouble digesting. Raffinose passes through the small intestine, undigested, and into the large intestines where your gut bacteria breaks it down. This produces gas that eventually you pass.

BUT...slowly incorporating more beans and lentils into your diet allows your system to get used to them, making them more easily digested, and decreasing gassiness. Beans and lentils have also shown to enhance overall gut health by improving intestinal barrier function and increasing beneficial digestive bacteria. If you are new to adding beans and lentils to your diet, start slowly to allow your digestive system to get used to them.

WHAT ARE BEANS AND LENTILS?

We're talking about things like chickpeas, beans (kidney, pinto, navy, black, pigeon and many, many more!), dried peas (split peas) and lentils. These are all the edible seeds of the plants in the legume family and are called "pulses".

Did you know that "legume" is the name of the whole plant including the leaves, stems, and pods. For example, a pea pod (think snap peas) is a legume but the pea inside the pod is a pulse.

Legumes and pulses are a nutritious staple of many diets around the world and have been cultivated by humans for approximately 6000 years!

SUPERFOOD?

I'm not a fan of the word *"superfood"* but when it comes to beans and lentils, I think it's appropriate. Check out all the nutrients these pulses are jam-packed with:

- Protein
- Fiber
- Folate
- Calcium
- Iron
- B vitamins
- Vitamin C
- Complex carbohydrates
- Potassium
- Antioxidants

Beans and lentils are digested slowly which gives a feeling of satiety. They also promote a slow burning, steady energy while the iron content helps transport oxygen through the body. This helps to boost energy and metabolism. The high amount of fiber is excellent for managing cholesterol, digestive health, regulating energy levels, as well as helping to stabilize blood glucose levels.

ENVIRONMENTAL HEROS!

Not only are they powerhouses in the nutritional department but did you know they are also good for the environment? Legume crops have a lower carbon footprint than almost any other food group. They are considered one of the most sustainable proteins in the world as they have the ability to enrich the soil, reducing the need for chemical fertilizers, and compared to other proteins, they need only one-tenth the amount of water to grow. They are also frost and drought resistant which makes them almost indestructible!

CANNED OR DRIED?

CANNED beans and lentils are definitely more convenient but also have a higher price tag. They are already soaked and cooked so are ready to be used in fresh or cooked dishes. Just rinse and go! Canned beans can be high in sodium so something to watch out for when purchasing. Be sure to rinse them well to remove as much sodium as possible but keep in mind they will have absorbed a lot of it. Look for low or no-sodium canned beans and lentils as a better alternative.

DRIED beans are much less expensive but involve some labour. They also take up less space in your pantry. Preparing them can be a bit time consuming as they require soaking and then simmering for up to a few hours, depending on the bean. I recommend preparing a whole bag at once and freezing whatever you aren't using. They freeze perfectly and are ready to use for whatever you are making! Lentils, on the other hand, don't require soaking therefore take less time to prepare.

LET'S BREAK DOWN THE COST DIFFERENCE

I'm using red kidney beans as an example.

These prices are an average and in Canadian dollars

COST

DRIED = $1.75 450g/1 lb

CANNED = $1.40 540 ml/18 oz

YIELD

DRIED 12 x ½ cup servings of cooked beans per bag

CANNED 4 x ½ cup servings per can

$ PER SERVING

Dried = $0.15 per serving

Canned = $0.35 per serving

So, if you are on a budget then dried beans are the way to go!

EASY WAYS TO ADD THEM IN

Another amazing thing about beans and lentils is how versatile they are! Because they have a sort of benign flavour, they get along well with virtually any ingredients, herbs, and spices. You can add them to almost anything!

- **Enjoy them as a quick salad topper** - Try roasting them with a bit of olive oil and your favorite spices to enhance their flavour!
- **Add them to soups** - Use them whole or pureed. Pureeing acts as a thickener.
- **Add to chili, curry, stew, and stir-fries** - You can use all beans for a meatless meal, or a combination of meat and pulses to cut down on your meat consumption and make it more nutrient rich.

- **Mash up** - chickpeas and mix with your favourite tuna salad ingredients for a vegetarian version!

- **Use them to make tasty and nutritious dips and spreads** - Hummus is the classic but you can puree any cooked beans or lentils, add some seasonings to make a dip or spread for a leafy green wrap!

- **Have them for breakfast with or without eggs** - Fry up some black beans with a bit of chili powder and top with cheese, salsa and avocado!

LET'S REVISIT CRAVINGS

At this point, if you are following The Program, you should find any cravings you had or have, are minimal. And if you do have them, they are nothing to be feared and can actually be your body giving you a heads up on its needs.

Cravings are just messages from the body. They are the body's way of communicating it's needs by associating the foods that can help get it what it needs.

It's important to remember your body is on your side and it's not trying to screw you over by craving.

If you are following the Food Plan, drinking the water, and taking the supplements, any cravings should be few and far between. And if they do pop up, it's usually just a matter of making a few tweaks.

LET'S TALK SUGAR:

The key to beating sugar cravings is to understand that it's not actually sugar people are addicted to; it's the high insulin levels needed to break it down that has you reaching for sweets.

WHY?

- Insulin is the hormone that allows your body to use glucose for energy. Glucose is a type of sugar found in carbs like fruits, vegetables, and naturally occurring sugar that your body uses for energy. After you eat food and your digestive system breaks it down, your pancreas releases insulin to help regulate your blood sugar.

- When you reach for the sweets or foods with high sugar content, your body can flood with too much insulin, which causes your blood glucose levels to drop. This creates a dip in energy and a desire for even more sugar.

- This can create a vicious cycle that makes taking sugar and carbs out of your diet a challenge.

WHY AM I CRAVING SO MUCH SUGAR IN THE FIRST PLACE?

LET'S BREAK IT DOWN:

1. **More is more:**

- When you have sugar, your body will immediately want more sugar. These cravings can be so intense that if you create a habit of having sugar at the same time every day, your body will begin to crave and expect it at that same time daily. This is also the reason you end up eating that whole box of cookies in one sitting!

THE FIX:

- Add some protein and fat.

- Making sure to add in healthy fats to your meals along with protein, will help to prevent any cravings along the way.

- But if you do find yourself indulging, you can neutralize sugar cravings by having some protein and fat with your sweet treat. For example, if you indulge in a cookie, you can cut the desire to eat another cookie by having a slice of cheese or a handful of nuts.

- The protein and fat will help neutralize the amount of insulin your body uses to break down the sugar and decrease your cravings, giving your will power a fighting chance to kick in and help.

2. **Dehydration is a factor:**

- When you are dehydrated and not picking up on the cues from your body to drink more, your body's next best bet is to crave foods with a high-water content, like fruit. Fruits are also sweet, so you may mistake your body's cue to consume more water and instead find yourself reaching for processed carbs and sugar.

- This is why you may hear the advice to drink a glass of water before you eat to satisfy your appetite. It doesn't satisfy your appetite, but if it's water that you actually need, you may realize you are not really hungry after all.

THE FIX:

- Drink more water.

- Sip water throughout the day, aiming for a minimum of 3.5 liters a day and even more on days you exercise or are more active.

3. **You are tired:**

- When you are tired, your body goes looking for a pick-me-up, and you may find yourself reaching for something sweet.

- The same thing happens around 3 or 4 p.m. each afternoon when the body is wired to take a drop in energy and slows your circadian rhythm. What your body is really looking for is a nap. (There are places in the world that do just that, and call it the siesta.)

- In our fast-paced, high-stress world, it's not always possible to take a nice afternoon nap, so the body goes looking for easy energy by way of higher sugar to pick it up and keep it going.

THE FIX:

- Make sure to keep up with your water because when you are dehydrated it can add to your tiredness.

- Be sure to eat all your meals and especially your snacks. This will help to avoid energy levels that dip when you go for long periods of time without eating.

- When it comes to meals and snacks, be sure to choose foods that have a high nutrient value to give the body the energy it needs. And be extra mindful of portions so you don't make the body work harder than it needs to.

- With a few adjustments, you can easily beat the need for sweets and stay on track to reach your goals and not be held captive by sugar cravings anymore!

LET'S TALK SALT:

When you crave sugar, it generally means that you need more water. When you crave salt, it generally means that the body is asking for more good fat.

When you are stressed, your body is revving high, you burn lots of calories, your brain works really hard and your body quickly gets depleted of its nutrients.

Periods of high stress can rapidly deplete your vitamin and mineral reserves. So, when you are stressed, your body is looking for more sustaining energy by way of good fat.

You don't have to be stressed for the body to need more good fat. Fat is essential for cellular function as well as brain and heart health. It also works like a transport system for your body to process and digest carbs and protein.

Your body would rather get that fat from the foods you eat than to utilize its emergency reserve. Without enough good fat coming in, your body will be reluctant to let go of the fat that makes you fat. So, one way you can speed up that fat loss process is to make sure you are getting lots of good fats in your meals and adding in an omega 3.

Now with that said there are times when the body craves salt because it is in need of actual salt, so be mindful to add salt to your foods or add in trace minerals. This is usually more of an issue in warmer months when electrolytes are a concern.

LET'S TALK TUMMY RUMBLINGS & HUNGER PAINS:

We are taught to believe if your tummy rumbles you must be hungry, when in fact that's not what the noise and rumblings are about. It's actually your body's natural MMC or Migrating Motor Complex. Your digestive system works like a self-cleaning oven where, in between processing and digesting food, it works to clear bacteria and food particles out of the small intestine.

Because we are eating so often during the day, the body is doing most of this work at night. As we move through the program, we will be phasing you into more natural patterns of eating which will be more in tune to your body's needs, which include the downtime it needs in between meals to self-regulate.

TO RECAP:

Cravings are nothing to stress about, though they can give you great insight into your body's needs. Usually, the smallest tweak or adjustments can make all the difference.

It's important to note it's not about controlling your cravings; it's about being in tune to them. As you progress through the program, you will become more in tune and able to differentiate between the body's needs and your wants.

You may also find yourself craving other kinds of foods and even specific foods. At the end of this process, your body will clearly let you know when it's hungry, what it's hungry for, and how much you need to eat.

It's actually super cool how in tune you can become to your body and it's needs.

Paying attention to those cravings can help you better meet your body's needs so that your body can focus on what you need to do to get and keep the scale moving.

WEEK 10 GUIDELINES: HIGHER PROTEIN & FAT REVAMP PART 2 AND INTRODUCING BACK ON TRACK

Continuing the Higher Protein and Fat tweak while Maximizing your efforts. This is also the week we introduce the concept of Back on Track (BOT).

For this week, we are continuing the Higher Protein and Fat Revamp tweak along with Maximizing your efforts day to day. This is also where we introduce the concept of Back on Track (BOT). Back on Track refers to following the original Food Plan as a method to help the body recover from/or get Back on Track after indulging in a way that causes the scale to be up or for you to feel "off". First, let's review the basics for the Higher Protein and Fat Revamp tweak.

RECAP OF THIS WEEK'S TWEAK

- **Breakfast** - still higher protein, ideally taking out any harder to digest carbs like bread, crackers, oatmeal's and go more for fish, eggs, yogurts, protein shakes, etc. If you haven't been having breakfast, now is a good time to add it in. Since we want dinner to be the smallest meal of the day, adding in breakfast can help make sure you aren't hungry in the evening.

- **Morning Snack -** can still be fruit but with added protein and fat. OR you can skip the fruit and just have protein and fat.

- **Lunch -** protein with veg and leafy greens. Eliminate any heavier carbs like potatoes, white rice, grains... except quinoa & black rice in small portions if needed.

- **Afternoon Snack (only one)** - There will only be one afternoon snack. You can combine the veg and nuts/seeds snack or see Week 9 Guidelines for other ideas/options.
- **Dinner** - Veg, protein and leafy greens. Please note the added carbs by way of the vegetables, which are now the star of the show at dinner. You can add in any heavier carb veggies here if you feel the need for them. This will help balance out the day of eating higher protein.
- **Refer to the Week 9 Guidelines for a review of the information.**

LET'S TALK BACK ON TRACK

Weekends, holidays and vacays can be tricky when it comes to staying on plan because we tend to be more off routine, making it a bit more difficult to follow the routine. Add in a long/holiday or celebratory day and it can make it even harder.

You may have heard me reference getting "Back On Track". BOT refers to getting back to the basics.

Back on Track is a technique you will use after indulging in or having an "off day", "off weekend", or even an "off week" of eating as you continue to work through the rest of the program to lose, and once you are in maintenance, to help maintain your weight.

Back on Track refers to the original Food Plan Formula, the same one you have been following these first few months of The Program.

The original Food Plan has now become a familiar routine for the body that will help it reset and catch up after any "off days."

THE METHOD OF GETTING "BACK ON TRACK":

- Protein for breakfast
- Fruit for snack
- Veg, protein and leafy greens for lunch
- Raw veg snack
- Nut and seed snack
- Protein and leafy greens for dinner

When eating "Back on Track," you want to eat all meals and snacks, but keep the portions on the smaller side.

This is NOT for the sake of eating less calories, but to help the body stay focused on getting rid of any backlog of food which is attributing to your weight being up.

You want to keep lunch and dinner light with more leafy greens and avoid any heavier carbs. You want to get in extra water.

You want to eat as early in the evening as possible. You want to help the body get a nice, deep sleep.

You want to move your body, go for a walk after dinner, have an epsom salt bath, and head to bed earlier. You also want to be as consistent as possible with the supplements.

If you get on the scale after indulging and your weight is up, it's important to understand that it is not real weight gain. Weight up is just from a backlog from hard to digest foods, salty food, and your body retaining water.

You will find after being "Back on Track" for a few days, your weight will drop right back down to where it was before you had your off day/s. And then you can carry on and pick up where you left off in The Program.

With that said, Back on Track is not always about the scale coming back down because sometimes your weight can be up for other reasons. In that case, you implement BOT until you "feel" BOT, which usually takes 1-3 days.

You may feel inclined to eat less or to skip meals and snacks after indulging thinking this will help you get ahead and Back on Track faster...it will not. Under-eating after over-indulging will only reinforce the need for the body to hold onto and store fat. It will also under stimulate your digestive system making it longer to get back on track.

- Keep in mind, Back on Track is NOT to be used unless you over indulged for a day or more.
- It is NOT meant to be used to manage day to day fluctuations on the scale or one "off" meal.
- It is best reserved for when you really go off the rails for a couple or more days. Not just one-off meal or indulgence.

How long you implement back on track depends on how off the rails you went, normally a day or two is plenty to help the body get back on track. Also, best to keep any indulgences to a minimum while looking to lose weight. Avoid the mentality of making this a lifestyle thing where you try to have your indulgences and lose weight too... Reserve Back on Track for the times you really need it.

Please take time to head over to the Facebook Group and watch the quick video that accompanies this post.

LET'S REVISIT BOWEL MOVEMENTS

We have talked a lot about bowel movements over the past few weeks.

When following the program, it's normal to have your bowel movements be all over the place, meaning every shape, size and consistency, as it's normal to have bouts of constipation and also normal to have loose bowel movements.

Constipation is usually the body responding to the changes you are making (change in routine of foods and change in type of foods) and also the body taking time to make improvements in digestion that can lead to improvements in regularity which is a good thing.

Loose bowel movements on the other hand are a normal and somewhat expected byproduct of the detox process we are piggybacking to lose weight. But can also be a sign of food sensitivities, which if you are keeping a journal, you should be picking up on.

If you have always suffered from bowel movement issues, you should see significant improvement by following the program. And once you are done helping the body focus on weight loss and are in maintenance, you will find your bowel movements will normalize giving you that S-Shaped Dr. Oz/Oprah bowel movements everyone strives for.

Your digestive health is directly associated with, and affects your bowel movements. Food goes in and it needs to go out. So, as you continue to focus on fat, loss here is what you can do, above and beyond following The Program, to help improve your bowel movements:

LET'S TALK CONSTIPATION:

THE BASICS:

- Drink lots of water
- Be sure to add leafy greens to meals
- Add in, and regularly take, the basic supplements: Omega 3, Vit D, Probiotic, and Calm magnesium.

In addition to what is listed above in regards to the basics, which all work together on Plan, we also suggest looking into adding:

PREBIOTIC:

- Prebiotic is food for your probiotic. Prebiotic does come in pill form but is best to get in a clear fiber.

- You can also increase your intake of prebiotic foods that help with digestion like: Onions, garlic, leeks, chickpeas, lentils, kidney beans, bananas, grapefruit, bran, barley, and oats.

DIGESTIVE BITTERS:

- Digestive bitters are herbs that support digestive function by stimulating bitter receptors on the tongue, stomach, gallbladder, and pancreas.

- They work to promote digestive juices such as stomach acid, bile, and enzymes, which help to break down food and assist in the absorption of nutrients.

- Look for Canadian bitters that come in drops you add to water.

- Take bitters about 20 minutes before a meal to signal your body to produce more saliva, bile, and stomach acid.

VITAMIN C:

- When taking higher doses of vitamin C, the extra or unabsorbed vitamin C pulls water into your intestines, which can help soften your stool.

- Take 30 mins before food in the morning, dose is dependent on the individual and can range from 90-2000 mg.

B COMPLEX:

- B12, B1 & B5 deficiency can cause constipation. If your constipation is caused by low levels of B's, increasing your daily intake of this nutrient may help ease your symptoms.

- B2 or B complex is part of the secondary supplements list I will be sending out in a few weeks.

- Not essential to weight loss, but it is key in supporting metabolic function, which can significantly help with weight loss, by helping to improve your energy.

- You may prefer to eat more foods rich in this vitamin rather than take a supplement.

EXAMPLES OF FOODS RICH IN B VITAMINS INCLUDE:

- Meat (red meat, poultry, fish)
- Beef
- Liver
- Trout
- Salmon
- Tuna fish
- Whole grains (brown rice, barley, millet)

- Eggs and dairy products (milk, cheese)
- Legumes (beans, lentils)
- Seeds and nuts (sunflower seeds, almonds)
- Dark, leafy vegetables (broccoli, spinach)
- Fruits (citrus fruits, avocados, bananas)

TRIPHALA:

- Used in Ayurvedic medicine for thousands of years. It's thought to support bowel health and aid digestion. As an antioxidant, it's also thought to detoxify the body and support the immune system.
- Triphala helps to keep the stomach, small intestine and large intestine healthy by flushing out toxins from the body.
- Triphala is available in supplement form, as a pill, and in powder form. The powder is meant to be dissolved in warm water and consumed as tea. It can taste bitter but can be mixed with honey or lemon without diminishing its effects.
- Triphala supplements have varying daily dosages based upon the manufacturer. It's important to follow package directions exactly.
- Triphala may be most effective when taken right before bed with a large glass of warm water.
- Some people prefer to take this supplement on an empty stomach, while others prefer to take it with food. Discuss these options with your doctor.

EXERCISE/MOVE YOUR BODY:

- Exercise helps constipation by lowering the time it takes food to move through the large intestine. This limits the amount of water your body absorbs from the stool.
- Cardio exercise speeds up your breathing and heart rate, helping to stimulate the natural squeezing of muscles in your intestines which helps to move stool out quickly.
- Something as simple as going for a walk after dinner can make all the difference when it comes to improving digestion.

TIME AND CONSISTENCY:

- It is important to note that in most cases the body just needs time to rewire how it has come to function over the years.
- The foods you are eating, and the overall structure of The Program will help from a baseline level to address constipation issues.
- Try to keep things routine and be patient with the process, but also don't suffer. Sometimes

you need to take something stronger like an over-the-counter laxative to help the body work through any backlog.

LET'S TALK LOOSE BOWEL MOVEMENTS:

Loose bowel movements can be unnerving but also a normal part of the process due to all the water you are drinking, leafy greens you are eating, as well as fiber rich foods like fruit and veggies which all contribute to a natural daily detox.

In most cases, it's nothing to be concerned about. However, here are some things you can do to address:

- Continuing to focus on digestive health. It can be a great idea to add in the prebiotic and bitters to help strengthen your digestive system.

- Keep a journal and record how you are feeling after eating meals and snacks as sometimes food sensitivities can pop up that can cause loose BM and discomfort.

- Dairy and gluten are the most common sensitivities, but it can come down to specific food choices like a kind of fruit for example, or even spicy food.

- Decrease calm magnesium. Although the calm mag is rarely the sole issue for loose BM, decreasing it slightly may help.

- If you are concerned about nutrient loss, rest assured, it's not a major concern when following the plan.

- You can add trace minerals to your water or add in a pinch of pink rock salt or Celtic salt to your warm water and lemon in the morning and/or water throughout the day.

- Add in Psyllium fiber. You never want to add in fiber while constipated as it can sometimes make the situation worse. It is however an excellent time to add in if experiencing loose bowel movements.

Psyllium is non-dependent and when added in, attaches itself to toxins stored in your fat cells and helps to draw them out. This can help make your bowel movements more binding and effective for fat loss.

- The soluble fiber also helps lower blood cholesterol levels and control blood sugar levels. You can also get this type of fiber from oats, barley, oranges, dried beans and lentils.

- Comes in pill or powder form. I personally like the pills.

- Take before bed or in between meals.

TO RECAP:

The body has been working hard to address digestive and BM issues. Given enough time, your body will continue to make significant improvements.

Although usually nothing to be concerned about, when it comes to BM issues, it is always recommended to check in with your doctor.

Some conditions including Crohn's disease, celiac disease, IBS, thyroid issues and medications can be the cause of loose BM, but if your changes in BM go hand in hand with following the program, chances are there is nothing to be concerned about and given the time, the body will sort out and address it on its own.

LET'S REVISIT SUPPLEMENTS

It is a great idea to revisit the supplement conversation since it is never too late to add them in and it is always a good idea to review them relative to where you are now in the program.

The following are basic supplements that, over the years, I have found helpful to aid in deficiencies in the body that may affect your ability to drop weight and/or can help speed up the process. Although they have many benefits, keep in mind these supplements are suggested because in my experience they can help with weight loss.

BASIC SUPPLEMENT LIST:

PROBIOTICS:

A probiotic is good bacteria added to your digestive system that helps promote a healthy immune system, but more importantly for our purpose, helps with weight loss by improving digestion.

Digestion is important for weight loss because if your body is unable to process food properly and get the nutrients your body needs, it will store fat to compensate or be reluctant to let it go.

- Probiotics come in pill, powdered, or liquid form.
- The probiotic added to foods like yogurt is usually not sufficient enough.
- I suggest looking for a "one a day" with higher potency. This helps minimize the number of pills you have to take each day. Probiotics come in a variety of different potencies and strains and also price ranges.

Look for a probiotic with a variety of strains, especially:

- L. acidophilus
- B. Longum
- B. bifidum
- L. rhamnose
- L. fermentum

DOSE

5-10 billion CFUs is an average potency. Follow the recommended dosage on your product's label.

WHEN TO TAKE

Take either on an empty stomach 30 mins before breakfast or with breakfast. The advantage of taking with or without food is debatable. You can also take it before bed. Whichever time you choose, try to be consistent with it. Avoid taking after a meal. Follow package directions for dose.

PLEASE NOTE

If you have SIBO you might be advised NOT to add in a probiotic. If unsure, always check in with your healthcare provider.

PROBIOTIC FOOD SOURCES

- Yogurt
- Kefir
- Buttermilk
- Some cheeses such as Gouda, Cheddar, Parmesan and Swiss
- Sauerkraut
- Kimchi
- Pickles that are naturally fermented like Strubbs. If they contain vinegar they aren't naturally fermented.
- Tempeh
- Miso
- Kombucha be mindful of sugar content

VITAMIN D, D3:

Vitamin D is beneficial for weight loss because it tricks the body into thinking it is summer year-round, eliminating the need for the body to hold on to the extra fat it feels inclined to store over the winter months. It is also essential in supporting the body's metabolism.

Low levels of vitamin D are often found in people who have weight to lose because when someone is lacking Vit D, the hypothalamus (the very small part of your brain that regulates hormonal functions, amongst other things) senses low vitamin D levels and responds by increasing body weight.

- Vit D comes in drops or pills. I like drops but pills work.
- Vit D2 is the vegan form
- Vit D3 is the most effective for raising levels as it absorbs better.
- It is better absorbed if taken with a meal that contains fat.

DOSE

600-2000 IU/day is the recommended dose range. Follow package directions for dose.

WHEN TO TAKE

Take with breakfast or lunch because taking it too late in the day can interrupt the body's production of melatonin and mess with your sleep.

OMEGA 3:

Without enough good fat in your diet your body can be reluctant to let go of your stored fat, so one way to speed up the fat loss process is to increase your intake of essential fatty acids.

30% of your diet should come from fat and ideally 10% of that should come from omega 3. The primary source of omega 3 is fish and unless you are eating a lot of it, it can be difficult for the body to get enough.

Best taken with food and ideally higher fat for best absorption. Because it can be hard to digest, you can divide the dose and take it at breakfast or lunch. Some find refrigerating or even freezing the capsules makes it easier to digest. Follow package directions for dose.

- Avoid taking before bed or before exercise as the increased activity can cause heartburn or reflux.
- Omega 3 comes in pill or liquid (oil). Both are equally good.
- If you don't like fish oil you can use vegan alternatives like a 3-6-9 combo.
- I would also look for a high potency one-a-day, again, to minimize the number of pills to take in a day.

DOSE

500-3000 mg per day is the recommended dose range. Follow the directions on your product's label for dose.

WHEN TO TAKE

Avoid taking before bed or before exercise as the increased activity can cause heartburn or reflux.

If you are on prescribed blood thinners, consult with a doctor before adding in.

CALM MAGNESIUM (MAGNESIUM CITRATE):

Although magnesium is responsible for over hundreds of actions in the body, it is important to us because, it not only helps to convert your foods into usable energy, it also helps calm the nerves and balance out cortisol levels (caused by stress.) This helps your body to relax, which can help with getting deep & REM sleep. Deep sleep is important because that is the kind of sleep you need for the body to best repair, rebuild, and detoxify.

- Calm Magnesium is also beneficial when it comes to addressing bowel movement issues, and in combination with omega 3 and a probiotic, can help make significant improvements.
- The most effective Calm Magnesium is in powdered form. The pill form doesn't have the same effect.

- It comes plain or flavored. The flavored ones have stevia added, but the benefit outweighs the effect of stevia if it keeps you taking it regularly.
- Take at night as directed before bed. You might need to play around with the dose to find what works for you. Start with the recommended dose and increase in small increments to get the desired effect.

DOSE

1-2 tsp per day is recommended. Follow the directions on your product's label.

WHEN TO TAKE

Take at night as directed before bed.

DIGESTIVE BITTERS:

If you have known digestive issues, or digestive issues that are as simple as getting bloated after eating raw veg or nuts and seeds, you may want to add in some digestive bitters.

- Digestive bitters help build up digestive enzymes that help with processing and getting nutrients from food.
- Bitters are better than taking digestive enzymes because they don't just help in the moment to process food, they also help to build up digestive enzymes that are normally created by eating raw foods.
- Bitters are also beneficial for anyone missing their gallbladder or suffering from acid reflux as they help to stimulate bile production.

DOSE

1-2 ml up to 3 times per day as directed on the label.

WHEN TO TAKE

Take between meals or 15 mins before meals.

PREBIOTIC WITH ADDED CLEAR FIBER:

If you have inflammation, digestive, or bowel movement issues, you might want to pick up a prebiotic with added clear fiber.

- Take with your Probiotic.
- Prebiotic is food for the probiotic and together can help improve digestion and bowel movements.

- It is being used more and more in gut therapy to address things like bowel movement issues, leaky gut, high histamine levels, inflammation, insulin resistance, Crohns, and Colitis.

DOSE

Follow directions on your product's label.

WHEN TO TAKE

Prebiotics can be taken any time of day.

COLLAGEN:

Taking collagen helps with tissue repair, improving the quality of hair and nails, but more importantly skin, which is important when it comes to weight loss.

- It's a non-essential protein naturally found in the body that depletes at a rate of 1% yearly after the age of 21.
- Collagen can also help with internal tissue repair and aid the body in making all the changes we are asking of it, as well as helping to maintain muscle mass.
- Most commonly sold in powder form and can be mixed into coffee, tea, water, oatmeal, yogurt etc.
- Collagen comes in either bovine sourced or marine sourced. Marine is better for skin and bovine is better for maintaining muscle mass, but both are effective. You can do your own research or speak to someone at your local health food store, to see which source and which brand is best for you.
- I personally use marine collagen. Specifically, the "Within Us TruMarine" brand and "Deep Marine" brand. But there are many quality brands to choose from.

DOSE

5-10g is the average dose recommendation. Follow the directions on your product's label.

WHEN TO TAKE

Collagen can be taken any time of day.

LET'S REVIEW THE SECONDARY SUPPLEMENTS

This list is for those of you who may be interested in taking things to the next level when it comes to your health and wellness.

MCT OIL:

MCT oil is a medium-chain triglyceride (MCT) which I started using about 15 years ago to help natural bodybuilders and professional athletes shed excess fat fast.

The reason why MCT oil is so great for fat loss is because it works like the old thermogenic supplements people used to take to burn fat, but without the harmful effects.

Unlike every other fat source that needs to be broken down, digested, and stored before it is of any use to the body, MCT oil is easily digested and sent directly to your liver where it has a thermogenic effect and the ability to boost your metabolism (the rate at which your body functions and burns calories).

MCT's are instantly utilized for fuel instead of being stored as fat, so it helps to calm the mind (since your brain is floating in cholesterol, it needs good fat for energy to function) but keeps the body revved up and working extra hard.

Look for MCT oil derived from 100% coconut oil, NOT coconut oil itself. Use as directed, although I suggest starting with 1 teaspoon and working your way up to a tablespoon per serving...to a max of 3 servings per day. Ideally, you can use it in the morning, around 3:00/4:00 pm, and then after dinner.

You can take it straight up, in oil form, add to coffee and shakes, or use as a dressing on salads.

DOSE

Use as directed, although I suggest starting with 1 teaspoon and working your way up to a tablespoon per serving...to a max of 3 servings per day.

WHEN TO TAKE

Ideally, you can use it in the morning, around 3:00/4:00 pm, and then after dinner.

Side effects can include digestive upset if you use too much too soon, so I cannot express how important it is to use less instead of more, and work your way up.

Please also make sure to continue taking your omega 3 supplements, as MCT oil is not an essential fatty acid.

ADRENAL SUPPORT:

Your adrenals are two nickel sized glands, just above your kidneys. Adrenals produce and control cortisol, the stress hormone. When you are stressed, your adrenals can produce too much cortisol or not enough. Cortisol is known as the stress hormone because of the body's stress response, although it is about more than just stress. Most of the cells in your body have cortisol receptors that use it for a variety of functions including: regulating blood sugar, reducing inflammation, regulating metabolism, and memory function.

We care about cortisol because too much or not enough, signals the need to store fat in the body.

WHO WOULD BENEFIT FROM ADRENAL SUPPORT?

Anyone who's been super stressed physically or mentally. Anyone with thyroid issues. Take as directed and be sure to check with your doctor.

DOSE

Follow the directions on your product's label for dosage.

WHEN TO TAKE

Take as directed and be sure to check with your doctor.

*Be sure to check in with your doctor if you are taking any antidepressant medications

TURMERIC:

The primary antioxidant in Turmeric the spice is curcumin, which is an anti-inflammatory. While increasing your intake of turmeric isn't a lone strategy for weight loss, it may help you address the inflammation associated with extra fat and help with metabolism.

Carrying extra fat creates low grade inflammation in the body that puts you at a higher risk of developing chronic diseases, like heart disease and type 2 diabetes.

Curcumin, which is an antioxidant in turmeric, suppresses the inflammatory messaging in many cells, including pancreatic, fat and muscle cells. This can help curb insulin resistance, high blood sugar, high cholesterol levels, and other metabolic conditions resulting from excess fat.

We care because when your body isn't fighting so much inflammation, it's easier to focus on weight loss.

Turmeric is a readily available spice, and adding it to your diet has no side effects unless you have an allergy, so it can easily be added to foods.

However, in order to get the amount of curcumin necessary to aid in weight loss you would have to use a lot of it. Therefore, if you want to experience the full effects, you need to take a supplement that contains significant amounts of curcumin.

WHAT TO LOOK FOR

Curcumin is poorly absorbed into the bloodstream, so it is better absorbed with black pepper. Black pepper contains piperine, which is a natural substance that enhances the absorption of curcumin by as much as 2,000%. The best curcumin supplements contain piperine, which substantially increases the absorption and therefore effectiveness.

DOSE

Follow the directions on your product's label for dosage.

WHEN TO TAKE

Follow the directions on your product's label.

NOTE: Turmeric, especially taken as a supplement, can interact with certain medications, so always consult your doctor when considering adding it to your diet. Turmeric can increase your risk of bleeding if you're on blood thinners, interfere with the action of drugs that reduce stomach acid and increase the risk of low blood sugar when taken with certain diabetes drugs. Turmeric is also contraindicated if you have gallstones or obstruction of the bile passages.

TRACE MINERALS:

Most of us are familiar with the vitamins we need and know how essential they are to our health and wellness. But even with taking a supplement, or choosing nutrient rich food, many people are not getting in enough trace minerals. Even though trace minerals are only required in small amounts, they are indeed essential. Not only for good health, but also weight loss.

THERE ARE TWO CLASSES OF MINERALS:

1. Major
2. Trace

Major minerals include: calcium, potassium, chloride, phosphorus, magnesium, sodium, and selenium. Trace minerals include chromium, germanium, manganese, rubidium, vanadium, cobalt, iron, molybdenum, zinc, copper, lithium, nickel, and silica.

Minerals are needed for important metabolic functions in the body and mineral deficiencies are involved in metabolic disorders that cause diseases including hypertension, headaches, depression, heart disease, insulin resistance, and obesity.

An important part of a successful correction of the metabolism to achieve weight loss is addressing the mineral deficiency and replacing them in the correct way. Most of the over the counter multivitamins do not have the required amounts of minerals, especially the trace minerals.

Because on the program you are drinking lots of water, adding in some trace mineral drops can be an easy and effective way to boost your metabolism. Adding in trace minerals can also help prevent low sodium levels caused from drinking too fast, drinking too much in a short period of time, and sweating.

DOSE

Follow recommendations on your product's label.

WHEN TO TAKE

Add to your water following directions on your product's label.

COQ10:

The primary role of CoQ10 is as an antioxidant. Your diet consists of antioxidants from a wide variety of sources, including fruits and vegetables.

The main source of dietary CoQ10 is from fatty fish such as mackerel, along with whole-grain foods. Your body also requires CoQ10 to produce energy from the carbohydrates and fat you eat in your diet.

CoQ10 assists in the production of energy by the cells. A deficiency can contribute to lower energy levels and a slower metabolism. Many people believe that CoQ10 production decreases with age, which can help explain one of the reasons why it can be harder to lose weight as you get older.

The CoQ10 can enhance healthy weight loss because it helps to support increased metabolic function. In addition, it can work to decrease body fat while boosting energy levels by maximizing your body's ability to convert food to fuel.

It's also great for the skin. Lack of CoQ10 results in decreased production of collagen and elastin. Collagen is important because it makes your skin firm, while elastin gives your skin flexibility. The loss of collagen and elastin causes your skin to wrinkle and sag.

DOSE

90–200 mg of CoQ10 per day is recommended, though some conditions may require higher doses of 300–600 mg. It is a relatively well tolerated and safe supplement.

WHEN TO TAKE

CoQ10 is fat soluble, so it should be taken with a meal containing fat so your body can absorb it. Also, taking CoQ10 at night may help with the body's ability to use and absorb it.

NOTE: Check with your doctor if you are on blood thinning or blood pressure medications.

B COMPLEX:

Vitamin B complex is a group of water-soluble vitamins, which play a very important role in maintaining the growth and the metabolism of cells in the body.

When it comes to weight loss, B12 is among the MOST IMPORTANT because it helps the body convert fats and proteins into energy. B12 is mainly found in red meat, chicken, fish, dairy and eggs.

A B Complex can help the body maintain sufficient levels of a variety of B vitamins so that it can efficiently burn carbohydrates, fats, and proteins and help the body maintain energy, stamina, and control appetite.

B-vitamins are water-soluble, meaning they are not stored in the body. Though they don't stick around long, B-vitamins are vital for supporting a variety of bodily functions. Most people get the right amount of B-vitamins through diet, but others may need to supplement these important vitamins through pills or shots.

Each B-vitamin supports different bodily functions, so your doctor will be able to pinpoint the supplements you need and help you decide between B12 vs. B-complex.

DOSE

Range is around 1.2mg. Follow directions on your products label.

WHEN TO TAKE

B vitamins can boost energy, so it is best to take them earlier in your day and with a meal. For dose, follow as directed.

L-THEANINE:

L-theanine is an amino acid found in both green and black tea leaves. It is also found in mushrooms, available in pill or tablet form.

It is thought to work by decreasing brain chemicals that contribute to stress and anxiety while increasing brain chemicals that encourage a sense of calm. L-theanine elevates levels of GABA, as well as serotonin and dopamine. These chemicals are known as neurotransmitters, and they work in the brain to regulate emotions, mood, concentration, alertness, and sleep, as well as appetite, energy, and other cognitive skills. Increasing levels of these calming brain chemicals promotes relaxation and can help with sleep. Some research also suggests that L-theanine may improve the function of the body's immune system and help to improve inflammation in the intestinal system.

There are no known side effects of taking L-theanine. It's safe to take the supplement and/or drink teas that contain L-theanine, though due to its calming effects, if you have low blood pressure, you may want to keep that in mind.

DOSE

Dose ranges from 100-400mg. Start with a smaller dose and work up.

WHEN TO TAKE

Follow the directions on your product's label.

As with all the suggestions, be sure to check with your doctor if you have any concerns.

LET'S TALK PEOPLE'S REACTIONS TO YOUR WEIGHT LOSS

Our Group Vibe Manager, Anna Blachuta, who is now down 90 lbs. in her journey, put together this post in the hopes of providing insight into how to manage comments and reactions to your ever-changing body.

First thing is first. You are doing this Program for you. Make sure you remember that each and every day. Let that be the driving force to get you to your "finally and forever". Whatever your end game is, it's yours. All of the work that you've put into yourself by doing this so far is amazing, and you deserve to be your best self! Nothing and nobody should get in the way of you achieving your goals.

Now that the world is slowly starting to open up and we are starting to see our friends and family again, we will have to also figure out how to navigate social situations. Handling people's reactions to your changing body is going to be a big part of that.

Always remember that no opinion but yours matters when it comes to your body and your choices. Whether you're bigger, smaller or anything in between, some people will always have something to say.

Positive or negative, you will feel like you are being treated in a different way than you ever have been in the past. These reactions can make you feel so many ways. There are times that people will be celebrating your successes, times where people can be uncomfortably negative or awkward, and even some times where others may try to sabotage your achievements (we all know one or two cookie-pushers!!).

I love the cheerleaders! They're a no brainer! Those are the friends and family you need to keep close. People say that it's not during the hard times when you know who your friends are, it's the great times. The positivity and light that comes from these people is gold - hang on to it for more motivation for you to keep pushing towards your goals!

There has been a lot of discussion recently with members having negative reactions about their weight loss from their loved ones. That negativity can be tough to handle. Even if you are a generally confident person, it can feel hurtful and unnerving.

There are many reasons why friends and family can have negative reactions to your weight loss.

- Jealousy
- Fear, shame
- Genuine concern
- People don't realize how impactful their words and opinions can be
- Social awkwardness, especially post pandemic
- Changing dynamic in a relationship (i.e., you're not the fat friend/sister/brother anymore)

The negative things people do may be different for everyone. Some examples of negative reactions include:

- Not saying anything or pretending not to notice your weight loss
- Asking if you're sick
- Questioning your portions, food choices, supplements, exercise routine…
- Saying things like, "enough already" and "You've lost too much weight - stop now!"
- Pushing unwanted food your way
- Judging you when you don't want dessert, a second portion, to finish your entire meal, etc.…
- Offering other weight loss programs/tips/advice
- Telling you that you were more fun (or cuter, or funnier…) when you were bigger

Sometimes, the negativity can even come from the people you trust the most in the world like your spouse or immediate family. Comments can be direct or indirect, like questioning portions or making small body-shaming jokes or remarks. This can be hurtful from anyone, but can be even more so for someone you are meant to trust or be vulnerable with. It can make you question what you're doing and everything you have done so far.

Here are some ideas to help you navigate these conversations:

1. **Be yourself!!** Such a cliché but, in my opinion, it is the best advice anyone can hear! You are on the road to your finally and forever - your life, thoughts, feelings and day to day will change. This is wonderful! No better time than now to practice being yourself and becoming your most confident you!

2. **Don't take it personally.** There are many people right now who have gone through their own dark times, including gaining a lot of weight, especially while trying to navigate through this global pandemic. They can be socially awkward because of the lack of social situations, and their own insecurities. It can be hard for them to handle your new positive outlook and healthy new look. This is them. Not you. Enjoy your new self and move on.

3. **React with kindness and stay calm.** Take a moment to carefully think about what you want to say, and breathe. Be polite, make sure you are expressing yourself in a respectful voice, and smile. Sometimes it's not worth it to stoop down to their level; it's nice to leave a negative situation feeling like the bigger person.

4. **Remember that no two situations are the same.** Think for a moment about how you want to handle this particular situation, because it may be different from others that you've encountered in the past.

5. **Diffuse the situation with humor**. It can sometimes release the tension of an awkward conversation.

6. **Talk to the person to tell them how you are feeling.** If you are not able to have a discussion in the moment, you can always take a step back, think about what happened, and pull the person aside to tell them how you feel. Be direct. Sometimes the conversation can be difficult but it can be just as difficult for you if you are constantly hearing negative comments from those you love.

7. **Don't overthink it.** If you've confronted someone about their behaviour and they do not respond well, remember that it is not your responsibility to change people. You've done the best you can to resolve the situation. Sometimes you have to accept that they have their own issues, realize that it is no fault of your own, and let them find their own solutions.

8. **If you need a cheerleader - reach out!** Our team and many of our past and current members are happy to help to give you the boost you may need!

Experiencing negative reactions is never fun, but remember that positive reactions are far more common. Be sure to make time for those positive people in your life. However, you want to navigate the negative situations is up to you, just be strong and remember that you are working towards becoming your best you!

FOOD FACTS - FOOD FOR A HEALTHY GUT

As soon as you began the Livy Method, you started improving your gut health. You did this just by implementing the food plan which naturally begins increasing the healthy bacteria in your digestive system and decreasing the unhealthy ones.

WHAT YOU ARE ALREADY DOING

- Eating lots of fresh fruits and veggies
- Regularly eating leafy greens
- Increasing healthy fats
- Eating raw nuts and seeds
- Taking apple cider vinegar
- Adding in pre & probiotic supplements
- Eliminating, or significantly decreasing, the amount of processed foods and sugar you are consuming

WHAT IS GUT MICROBIOME?

Microbiome is a word we are hearing more and more these days. It's popping up everywhere but do you know what it means?

Microorganisms or microbes are microscopic living things like bacteria, viruses, and fungi. The gut microbiome refers to the microbes found in your digestive system and can affect many aspects of your health. Did you know there are about 100 trillion bacteria, good and bad, that live in your digestive system?

"Altogether, these microbes may weigh as much as 2–5 pounds (1–2 kg), which is roughly the weight of your brain. Together, they function as an extra organ in your body and play a huge role in your health." - *healthline.com*

We all have healthy and unhealthy microbes in our gut but when things get out of whack and the unhealthy ones start to take over, it can have a negative impact on your health. An unhealthy balance can contribute to weight gain, increased blood sugar levels, chronic inflammation, decreased cognitive function, heart disease, as well as many other areas that are currently being studied. Many things, including the foods we eat, can impact the balance of bacteria found in the digestive tract.

HOW CAN I CONTINUE TO IMPROVE OR SUPPORT MY GUT HEALTH?

If you want to go further in improving your gut health, or supporting what you've already done, there are some specific foods that can help you level up your gut microbiome. These foods help to increase healthy bacteria and decrease the ones we want less of.

HERE'S A FEW THINGS YOU CAN DO, OR DO MORE OF!

EAT A VARIETY OF FOODS, ESPECIALLY PLANT FOODS - Different foods lead to a more diverse microbiome. Maybe it's time to start experimenting with different foods you have never tried before! Also decreasing meat consumption and replacing it with plant-based proteins can help increase healthy bacteria in the gut.

EAT CRUCIFEROUS VEGGIES! - So many benefits to these super veggies including healing your gut! High levels of prebiotic fibers and the powerful antioxidant, sulforaphane help to increase the healthy bacteria in your gut. Eating a variety of these veggies raw, or cooked, contributes to a diverse microbiome.

EAT FERMENTED VEGETABLES - sauerkraut, kimchi, miso, tempeh and naturally fermented pickles (found in the refrigerated section and should say "fermented". Not the same as pickled pickles found in the aisles). Fermented foods contain more lactobacilli which is a type of bacteria that can benefit the health of your gut.

EAT OTHER FERMENTED FOODS - Yogurt, kefir & kombucha. When it comes to yogurt, look for "contains live active cultures" and avoid products with high amounts of sugar.

EAT FOODS THAT ARE HIGH IN PREBIOTIC FIBERS - Apples, asparagus, bananas, barley, dandelion greens, garlic, leeks, oats, onions & seaweed to name a few.

INCORPORATE WHOLE GRAINS - Whole grains contain lots of fiber and nondigestible carbs that make their way to the large intestine promoting the growth of beneficial bacteria.

EAT PULSES - Remember our friends beans and lentils? They are also high in prebiotic fiber and help promote a healthy digestive system!

THE BOTTOM LINE IS...

You are already doing wonders for your gut microbiome just by following the plan. These are just some tips for those of you looking to level up or maybe just make some improvements. Every little bit adds up!

LET'S REVISIT LEAFY GREENS

Great for your brain, your bones and weight loss.

Leafy greens are an ideal addition to meals because they are not only packed with tons of nutrients that are great for your health and cellular function, but they also help the body process food through your digestive system, which is needed for weight loss.

High in fiber and water content, leafy greens help to keep you more satisfied by feeding into your satiety hormones which keeps you feeling more satisfied on smaller portions.

Increasing leafy greens can also play a role in keeping blood sugar levels stable by feeding into GLP-1 (Glucagon-Like Peptide-1) which is a hormone produced in your gut which helps to regulate your appetite.

Darker leafy greens are also rich in sulfur-containing compounds that support your body's detoxification process.

Plus, all of the changes you have been making in your diet can affect your bowel movements. Leafy greens provide the roughage your body needs to keep you regular throughout this process.

Leafy greens can be added to meals raw, like in a salad, but given the colder temps this time of year, you might find them more appealing cooked or sautéed and/or added to soups, stews & stir-fry dishes.

The general rule is...if it's green and leafy it works!

However... Cabbage, Brussels sprouts, and bok choy (among others which are listed in the Grocery List) which are cruciferous vegetables can also be used as leafy greens on plan.

Cruciferous vegetables are a major source of glutathione. Glutathione is an antioxidant in your body that is involved in tissue repair and boosting your immune system. (See Andrea's post on Food Facts on Cruciferous veg for more)

If you are not a fan of eating your leafy greens, it is still key to get them in.

You don't have to be fancy about it or get in a huge variety. It's also not a big deal if you are a bit hit and miss getting them in, as long as you are mindful to be as consistent as possible. But with that said, if you are looking to maximize your efforts...load them up!

Although they are suggested at lunch and dinner, they can also be added to breakfast and even your snacks moving forward

WEEK 11 GUIDELINES: PERSONALIZING THE FOOD PLAN

This week has you taking what you have learned and tweaking the Food Plan to suit your body's changing needs day to day while helping it to focus on fat loss.

This is an exciting place to be in your Weight Loss journey!

You have followed through and done a lot of work, not only to address why your body was feeling a need to store fat, but to help your body be as healthy as possible.

I have been saying all along that counting calories and weighing and measuring your food is not normal. Neither is the formula we have been using; forcing the body to eat certain foods at certain times has been the way we got the body's attention and helped it to focus on fat loss.

We used the formula in the beginning to give the body what it needed so it no longer felt the need to store fat. Then we used that formula to get the body to focus on and go into detox as much as possible for as long as possible, when fat loss wasn't yet a priority for the body.

Then, as fat loss became more of a priority, we used the formula to feed into and support the nice, high metabolism you have created throughout the Process, so your body can function at a more optimal level.

At this point, your body doesn't want the fat it was storing any more than you do, and it is more than happy to get rid of it, so you are going to use that to your advantage.

We will continue to use the original Food Plan formula when you need to get "Back On Track" after having an off day/s or indulging in foods that make you feel off. But unless you are in that situation, the formula is no longer needed.

THIS BRINGS US TO WEEK 11: PERSONALIZING THE FOOD PLAN.

**This stage of the program is the most work because it's about having faith in all the hard work you have done and the foundation you have built. **

It's also about RELENTLESSLY MAXIMIZING everything you can, and need to do, to keep the body focused on fat loss until you reach your goal.

WHAT DOES PERSONALIZING THE PLAN LOOK LIKE?

You are still following all of the basic guidelines like eating higher protein at breakfast, not going longer than 3.5 to 4 hrs. without eating, still making sure to drink your water, take your supplements and Maximize your efforts. The difference is you will be making your food choices based on the following:

1. **WHEN TO EAT** - You will still be checking in at each meal and snack time: breakfast, snack, lunch, snack, snack, dinner.

   • Before every meal and snack time, ask yourself if you NEED to eat, COULD eat or SHOULD eat. You still don't want to go longer than 4 hours without eating. That is where "should I eat" comes in. If not hungry, just have a token amount and check in at the next meal or snack time.

   • Keep in mind that hunger levels naturally fluctuate daily, meaning one day you might feel hungry every half hour and the next day, 3 to 4 hours will go by without being hungry.

   • Trust your mind-body connection and understand that the body knows best and it will let you know when it's hungry.

2. **WHAT TO EAT** - (while still following the Guidelines) When you are hungry ask yourself, what exactly am I hungry for and what's the best choice for me to Maximize my efforts.

   • You still want to choose your meal and snack options from the same kinds of foods you have been eating all along. But rather than eating specific foods at specific times, you can now make your choices based on what's most appealing in the moment when you are hungry. For example, you may choose to have fruit in the afternoon and nuts in the morning.

3. **HOW MUCH TO EAT** - Continue being super in tune and mindful about portion sizes, keeping in mind you are still looking to lose weight.

   • You want to continue to eat "just enough".

   • You DO NOT want to be matching your hunger levels. You want your body to keep momentum and focus on detox and fat loss, rather than processing and digesting food. Smaller portions are better for digestion and keep the food moving in and out.

- Smaller portions also help lower insulin levels so that you feel more satisfied on less, while keeping energy levels maintained.

GUIDELINES:

- Check in at every meal and snack time. Try not to let more than 3.5 - 4 hours max go by without eating.

- You are NOT introducing any "new foods". You are sticking with the same kinds of foods you have been eating. For example, no bars or muffins, and still no pasta.

- Breakfast is still an option, but always a benefit. If you do have it, still go with higher protein.

- Morning snack is your choice and can be optional, depending on if and when you had breakfast.

- Lunch can be your choice and more of a snack size. You can add back in the heavier carbs, but only as needed while still trying to lose.

- Leafy greens are still a benefit, especially if BMs are still an issue.

- Afternoon snacks you can have 1 or 2, or you can skip snacks depending on lunch and dinner times and your hunger levels (ideally no longer than 3.5 4 hours between eating).

- Dinner should be the smallest meal of the day, and can be more of a snack or snack-sized portion, and/or you can skip if not hungry. Avoid heavier carbs at this meal, unless needed.

ALWAYS MAXIMIZING:

- Water intake
- Supplements
- Being in tune to hunger levels
- Being in tune with portion sizes
- Managing stress levels
- Using your energy, being more active
- Working the parameters of the program. Meaning, still eating protein for breakfast and not eating or snacking late at night.

TO RECAP:

The purpose is to transition the body into a style of eating more conducive to helping it focus on fat loss, while feeding into its need to function more efficiently and at optimal levels.

At this point, the body wants the fat gone as much as you do, which means you no longer need to manipulate it into focusing on fat loss. In a sense, it means that day in and day out, you are Maximizing everything you can do to help the body continue getting rid of fat.

People can be reluctant about this phase because they feel there is less structure. But the reality is, it is just as structured, if not more so, since you will be checking in at every meal and snack time.

It's also more work because it's about bringing everything you have learned over the past few months together and not only implementing it, but Maximizing it.

TO SIMPLIFY WEEK 11:

The biggest change is; you no longer need to force the body to eat token amounts when you are not hungry unless 3.5 to 4 hours have gone by since you last ate. Pretty much everything else is the same, since you are still looking to lose weight by following the Guidelines & Maximizing.

Remember, the goal is for you to not only lose your weight in a healthy and maintainable way, it's to eventually wake up, look good, feel good, and just go about your day making good food choices. The goal is to get out of the weight loss game, lose your weight, and move on.

This stage of Personalizing The Plan will not only help you to continue to drop fat, it will set you up to be able to move on and have your food choices be based on your body's needs, rather than its wants. It's to have you move forward in life and never look back, and to give you the tools you need to forever be in tune so that you never need to lose weight again.

We are not done yet! The goal is to finish as strong as you started.

Please take time to head over to the Facebook Group and watch the quick video that accompanies this post.

FAQS WEEK 11

Here are some common questions we get asked about Week 11.

1. **Can we add bread and pasta back in?**

   - Keep in mind, some people have been eating bread and pasta all along and losing weight just fine. It's always been a choice. But make no mistake, it is not Maximizing your efforts while looking to lose.

   - If you still have weight to lose, it's best to keep them to a minimum.

2. **Is it better to skip lunch or dinner?**

   - You don't want to be skipping any meals "just because". If you are not eating a meal, it would be because you are not hungry for it. And even then, you need to take into account if you should eat based on the 30 minutes to 3.5 hours between meals and snacks.

3. **If I skip meals and snacks will my body go into starvation mode?**

   - Not if you are following the 30 minutes to 3.5 hours between meals and snack rule. If you go past 3.5 hours and you are not hungry, then this is a case of where you "should" eat at least a token amount of the next meal or snack.

4. **Can I have a protein shake for my lunch or dinner?**

   - Best to use at breakfast or snacks, but if you do use at lunch or dinner then you are still to include the protein, veg and greens. Although you can add a bit of fruit like you would at a meal, you still want to include the components of protein, veg and greens in your shake.

5. **Are we still making meals nutrient rich?**

   - Absolutely, nothing changes there! Be sure to add good fats to your meals and make them as nutrient rich as possible

TO RECAP:

You are very much still following The Plan, the only real thing that changes is you no longer have to eat token amounts if you are not hungry unless it's been 3.5-4 hours since you ate last, and you have a bit more flexibility in your food choices.

PERSONALIZING THE PLAN IS NOT EATING OFF PLAN

Let me say that again.

Personalizing the Plan...is not eating off Plan.

Week 11 is just another tweak like any other week on The Program. Be sure to read over the Guidelines...a few times.

Also, be sure to review the HUNGER & MAXIMIZING Posts and Videos as suggested for each new week.

We are assuming you are not done losing weight...so each week is still all about losing and Maximizing your efforts...right to the very end.

Now is NOT the time to do your own thing, if you are looking to capitalize on these last few weeks... be all in and follow the Program as designed.

BREAKFAST:

- You can skip it, though it is still a benefit to go higher protein. Go for the biggest bang for your buck.

- You can have protein shakes but it's still ideal to eat your food.

- You can add fruit, but be mindful of breakfast being higher in protein.

MORNING SNACK:

- You can skip it if you had breakfast and are not hungry for it. As long as you aren't going longer than 3.5 4 hours since breakfast.

- Otherwise, go by how you feel and choose something within the guidelines from what you have been eating these past few months.

LUNCH:

- Be sure to include the components of protein, veg and leafy greens adding in heavier carbs as needed.

- There is no star of the meal...add the components and then go by how you feel. If you are craving more protein, eat more protein.

- Lunch is still the place to add in heavier carbs as needed.

FIRST AFTERNOON SNACK:

- You can skip it if not hungry for it, still being mindful of the time since you last ate.

- Otherwise, snacks can be your choice from the same kinds of foods you have been snacking on thus far. Raw veg, fruit, nuts or seeds, yogurt for example.

SECOND AFTERNOON SNACK:

- Skip it if not hungry but be sure not to let more than 3.5 4 hours go by without eating.
- Ideal to still have nuts and seeds at that time if hungry but you can also choose from the pool of other snacks you have been eating these past few weeks.

DINNER:

- Should be the smaller meal of the day.
- No star of the meal but still ideal to include protein, veg and leafy greens.

EXTRAS TO KEEP IN MIND:

Still ideal to eat dinner as early as possible Still ideal to not eat after dinner

Still ideal to minimize breads and pastas

Still Maximizing

MAXIMIZING YOUR PERSONAL PLAN

Now that you have had some time to work on Personalizing The Food Plan with Week 11, it's time to take things to the next level. While Personalizing the Food Plan, you are still following the basic guidelines of The Plan.

For example, still having higher protein at breakfast, still being mindful to add in leafy greens when you can, keeping food nutrient rich, and still trying not to eat too late in the evening.

Along with Maximizing all the things you can do to keep the body focused and ready for "detox", you are checking in with yourself throughout the day to be sure you are in tune with your body's needs in the moment.

CONTINUING TO:

- Be mindful when you are hungry and when you are not.
- Be mindful of making the best choice in the moment.
- Be mindful of portion sizes, making sure to eat enough but not match hunger levels.
- Drink your water.
- Be consistent with supplements.
- Manage stress levels.
- Move your body.

LET'S TALK: NEXT LEVEL

When it comes to weight loss, there is a difference between eating well, eating better, and eating in a way that is conducive to weight loss. Some foods are easier to digest than others which is something to keep in mind when looking to lose weight and being in tune. In understanding how your body processes and digests certain foods, you can take things to the next level with your food choices.

For example:

Juice...and other liquid nutrients hit your body fast...making this an issue because it's hard to control Insulin levels

- Juice can be great in the summer when it's super hot or when you overexert yourself so much you need to replenish your glycogen (energy) stores fast. (Note these occasions are rare).

Fruits... are easiest to digest so perfect when you need quick and easy energy.

- Fruits are also nutrient rich and high in fiber. If you are not looking for quick energy or are mindful of spiking insulin levels, it's a good idea to pair with protein & fat to neutralize.

Veggies... are harder to digest than fruits but are good for stimulating the digestive system and have a high nutrient value.

- They are also great for increasing digestive enzymes and serve as an energy food, giving the body the carbs it needs without spiking insulin in the way fruit can.

Nuts and Seeds...take 2-3 hours to digest.

- High in protein and fat, they can help give you more sustaining (lasting) energy.

Fish and seafood... is easy to digest protein, which can take 40 minutes 1.5 hours.

Chicken/poultry takes approximately 2 hours

Eggs take around 45 minutes

Beans and legumes take approximately 1.5 - 2 hours

Red meat and pork...take the longest and can take 5+ hours (hard to digest but also high in B vitamins, so good to have when you crave).

Dairy...can take just as long as meat. (Dairy can be hard to digest, especially if you are sensitive to it, which is why it can be beneficial to limit).

EXAMPLES OF HOW YOU CAN USE THIS INFORMATION TO YOUR ADVANTAGE

1. **"I'm feeling low on energy and need a quick snack, so I'll grab some nuts"**

   Nuts take 2-3 hours to break down, whereas fruit takes 20-30 minutes. So, if you are looking for quick and fast energy, fruit is a better choice than nuts.

   Nuts are hard to digest, which is why in the beginning of The Program, we added them as a second snack in the late afternoon, to purposely make the body work hard and keep you more satisfied longer. So, when grabbing something easy and looking for more sustained, longer lasting energy, you may want to have some nuts.

2. **You are going out for a night on the town or a late event**

   Instead of having something like steak, which is harder to digest, have fish or seafood, which is much faster and easier to digest. That will give you the energy you need to enjoy your night out without interrupting your sleep later.

   These are things to keep in mind when wanting to take your eating to the next level, Maximize weight loss results, and have a deeper level of understanding as to why I suggested eating certain foods at certain times. Also, why eating hard to digest food in the evening makes no sense. There is a lot to be learned from many angles when it comes to making your food choices.

LET'S TALK: TOP TIPS FOR GOOD DIGESTION:

1. **Check in at scheduled meal and snack times.**

   Life can get busy and it's easy to get sidetracked and forget to eat. Until it becomes second nature, it's a great idea to check in on yourself.

   Although on Plan, it is important to be consistent with your food choices because it has a regulating effect on your digestive system. It's also important to allow your Migrating Motor Complex to kick in and do its work in between meals.

   Knowing when you are hungry and when you are not is key.

2. **Be conscious of what you eat and your portion sizes.**

   If you are still looking to lose, it's still key to be mindful of portions.

   Too much sugar or too large of a portion stimulates the pancreas to release more of the hormone insulin, which signals weight gain. Also, it does stress the body out when you indulge. For example, eating too much not only slows the weight loss process, it's also the number one cause of indigestion. Although, it's no big deal since you can always get Back on Track.

3. **Chew your food completely and don't talk while eating.**

   Incomplete chewing and talking while eating can cause premature swallowing. Our digestive systems are not designed to digest large pieces of food. When we put large pieces in our stomach, it can lead to incomplete digestion and digestive discomfort.

4. **Relax while eating your meal.**

   This may seem super simple, but many of us are always on the go and always on the clock rushing through everything we do.

   Eating when you are rushed increases your stress and slows down the digestive process. Try to create a calm atmosphere when eating.

5. **Practice good posture.**

   This is key especially with your ever-changing body, just from a structural point of view and making sure muscles are supporting proper alignment.

   When you slouch or hunch over, extra pressure is put on the digestive organs in your abdomen. This extra pressure can cause poor digestion. You should practice sitting with your shoulders back and your chin tucked in. This will allow more room for the digestive organs and will help improve digestion.

6. **Don't eat late at night.**

This is pretty standard on Plan but worth repeating why. Our bodies, including our digestive system, slow down in the evening hours as it gets ready to rest and rejuvenate. When we put food into our stomach at these late hours, there are not enough digestive enzymes to properly digest it. This undigested food sits in your stomach and will often disturb your sleep and prevent the body from focusing on detox.

7. **Take a brisk walk after eating.**

Increased physical activity after a meal actually helps jump start your digestive system and increases the production of digestive enzymes. This will lead to more complete digestion of your food.

8. **Try a spinal twist.**

Spinal twists allow excess toxins in the digestive system to be released, which has a calming effect. While in a cross-legged sitting position, slowly turn to the right and hold while taking 5 deep breaths, then repeat this process on the left side.

9. **Avoid ice cold drinks while eating.**

Although a nice cold glass of water can be refreshing in the warmer months, ice cold drinks can slow down the digestive process.

Think of it as putting ice on a muscle. The muscle stiffens and does not function as well. Warm or room temperature water or teas will encourage proper digestion even in the warmer months.

Now, this isn't to say you can't drink cold water while eating, just be in tune to how it may be affecting your digestive system in the moment.

REMEMBER:

These tips are not meant to stress you out or to complicate the process. I'm putting out this info for those interested in Maximizing their efforts and taking things to the next level.

Rest assured, you are doing enough by being mindful with the Process and following along as designed.

We hope you are enjoying this week of Personalizing the Food Plan and trying to have fun with it as you work to take things to the next level.

LET'S TALK AVOIDING WEIGHT GAIN

With many of you expressing concern about gaining weight back...and rightfully so, given past experiences, I thought it would be a great idea to talk about how not to gain weight back after putting all of your time and energy into losing it.

First, it's key to understand that the way you have gone about losing weight with this Process is different from any past attempts at fat burning.

When you burn your fat off by restricting energy foods or starving and depriving your body, you leave the body with no choice but to burn its stored fat for fuel.

Although it's effective for weight loss, it also immediately reinforces the need for your body to hold onto and store fat.

Simply put, if you use your body's stored fat for energy as a method for weight loss (fat burning), your body will store it all back plus more the first chance it gets, every single time ...and it will do so thinking it's doing you a favour!

Which is why you can lose weight with a fat burning diet, but you can't maintain the loss after you go back to normal eating.

With this Process, because you have addressed the body's need to store fat and have helped the body drop fat in the healthiest of ways, that's not really a concern.

However, there are 2 main reasons why someone might gain weight back after this Process that you need to be mindful of.

NOT PUTTING TIME INTO MAINTENANCE

- Maintenance is key. You have got to give your body time to get used to functioning at your new weight. You want your new weight to become your new norm / set point.

- Even though you may have hit your goal and are done losing, your body is not done solidifying the weight you have lost.

- Things like metabolism, blood flow, body temp and hormones are just a few of the things the body will need to address & adjust to be able to stabilize at your new weight.

- There are 2 phases to Maintenance. The first is going to last 2-3 months, where you are mindful to follow your Personalized Plan and not add in things that will stress the body out. If you do indulge, you will simply implement Back On Track.

- The second phase is where you go live your life and eat according to your body's fluctuating needs day to day. When you indulge, you will use Back on Track, but otherwise, you will just be waking up and going about your day being mindful of your food choices and how you feel.

Mindfulness moving forward is all you will need to be able to live a worry-free life when it comes to your weight.

This is also where the concept of "Check Yourself Before You Wreck Yourself" comes in. You don't gain 10 or 20lbs without noticing. Continue to be mindful and when you notice, simply check yourself and implement BOT.

NOT ADJUSTING TO SITUATIONAL CHANGE

- For example, losing your weight at home where your routine, environment and stress levels are different than if you went back to work. The situation being you were at home all day and now you are at your place of work.

- Another example of this would be to have a change in job, where your stress levels are different. Helping the body manage new stress by bumping up omega 3, adding in MCT oil or being mindful to get to bed earlier to adjust to your new schedule, are a few examples of what you can do to help minimize the impact of situational change.

- It's key to help the body adjust and adapt to change. Change in environment for example; needing more water in a dryer environment than you are used to. Adjusting to stress as noted above, or even a change in the times you are able to eat. For example, having more business meetings or a job that restricts when you can eat.

- The goal is to minimize the impact on the body by helping it adjust to physical or emotional stress/change.

I'm going to add a 3rd element to be mindful of, which is seasonal change.

SEASONAL CHANGE

- This one is all about not forcing yourself to eat salads when you are craving heavier carbs. In the cooler months, for example, be sure to be in tune to your body's needs. Heavier carbs, fatty meats, along with hot and spicy foods are more appealing for a reason. They help to create heat in the body which helps to eliminate the need for the body to store extra fat to keep you warm.

- Alternatively, be sure to decrease the heavier carbs & bump up fruits and cooling foods like salads and veg in the warmer months.

- Try to eat a seasonally sourced diet or incorporate seasonal foods WHEN possible.

THINGS TO AVOID TO PREVENT WEIGHT GAIN:

- Making a habit of going all day without eating. If this happens every now and then, it's no big deal. But if you make it a habit (like for weeks & months) ... the body will pick up on this and start storing fat.

- Trying not to eat all day in anticipation of a bigger meal later in the day. This only reinforces the need for fat when you starve the body followed by overeating, which leads to increased insulin levels & signals weight gain.

- Not eating the next day after indulging. Although you may not feel like eating much after a day of indulging, it's key to help stimulate the digestive system to help get rid of any backlog.

- Falling back into old habits like thinking less is more and trying to control your body instead of being in tune to it.

- Over exercising and not giving the body enough rest in between workouts can lead to the body feeling a need to store fat to compensate.

- Not prioritizing your body's needs like managing stress and getting enough sleep.

- Not replenishing the body or helping it heal after illness. For example, not taking probiotics after antibiotics or pushing it to recover too soon.

- Using artificial sweeteners that can lead to insulin resistance.

- Not drinking enough water. Although you don't need to be drinking as much water, once you lose you do want to be mindful of being hydrated so your body can function properly.

- Not being mindful of your body's ongoing and ever-changing needs.

As you can see, easily maintaining your weight truly is about being mindful and continuing to be in tune to your body's needs while you navigate and enjoy life.

It's not as hard as you think and a little effort goes a long way in terms of living a worry-free life when it comes to your weight.

Please take time to head over to the Facebook Group and watch the quick video that accompanies this post.

WEEK 12 GUIDELINES: MAINTENANCE AND MINDFULNESS

This week we will be having discussions on moving forward after you are done losing and how to proceed if you have more weight to lose after the Group is done.

As we enter the final week of the winter session, it's time to talk about Maintenance for those of you who have reached your goal, or are getting close.

To be clear, Maintenance is for those of you who are done losing & are no longer working towards getting the body to drop more fat.

**For those of you still looking to lose, continue with your Personalized Food Plan and later this week we will be discussing next steps for continuing your weight loss journey. **

There are two stages of Maintenance:

STAGE 1 MAINTENANCE: LASTS FOR 2 TO 3 MONTHS

This is when you have reached your goal and are now looking to solidify the weight you have lost so you can easily maintain it moving forward.

During this phase, you might look forward to adding back in all the foods you have gone without over the past few months.

HOWEVER, you still want to be mindful of choosing foods that will challenge the digestive system and cause stress internally.

This is even more important with all the added stress you may be under these days. The goal for the first stage of Maintenance is to give your body time to adjust and get used to functioning at your new weight. In other words, the goal is for your new weight to become the new normal for your body.

- During this FIRST Maintenance stage you will continue with your Personalized Food Plan but in a more relaxed manner because you are not looking to lose weight.
- Every now and then you can add in some of your old favorites but be sure to get "Back on Track" and help your body balance it out.
- It's best to keep any indulgences few and far between for the next few months.
- Just because the body is done dropping fat, doesn't mean it is done doing the work to support it.

SIDE NOTE:

For anyone concerned about loose skin, this is a great time to help that along.

Try dry brushing, adding in collagen & using natural oils and creams, as the skin takes twice the amount of time to regenerate around your new frame. Your skin cells will be regenerating as your body continues to work on addressing any issues above and beyond weight loss.

With your body now minimizing its focus on fat loss, it can allocate resources to other areas of the body when it comes to repairing, rebuilding, regenerating, and rejuvenating.

You have done a lot of work up until now. Your body is now working harder and will continue to do so, so the goal is to keep it working at these optimum levels.

STAGE 2 MINDFULNESS: THIS WILL BE ONGOING

This is when you are not giving much thought to what you are eating or not eating, and you start to move on and live your life by being in tune to your body's needs.

- You should now have faith in all your hard work by being able to wake up and go about your day, making good food choices in the moment.
- You should be in a place where your internal dialogue, and that space in your brain reserved for obsessing about what you eat and don't eat, is non-existent or getting close to it.
- This is where you move on and enjoy your life without worrying about what you are going to eat or not eat, or having to lose weight.

But, with that said, this is also where you implement the concept of "Check Yourself Before You Wreck Yourself".

CHECK YOURSELF BEFORE YOU WRECK YOURSELF

Although you have lost weight in a healthy way that has you in tune to your body's needs, it's not a magic pill.

Moving forward, you will always need to be mindful of the choices you make, understanding how your choices will affect your body, and then self-correcting, balancing out, and getting Back On Track to minimize the effect.

I've been able to easily maintain my weight for over 25 years. My weight has fluctuated up and down naturally and sometimes more than others, but for the most part, it's just a matter of going by how I feel.

If I make crappy food choices, I feel crappy, then I just get Back On Track. I never indulge without understanding how I will feel after. This may seem like work but after a while, it just becomes second nature.

Maintenance really is as simple as that.

You want to allow your body the time it needs to adjust to its new weight and continue to be in tune to your body's needs, being mindful of the messages you are sending and receiving.

LET'S TALK WATER AND SUPPLEMENTS

Once you reach Maintenance, you can re-evaluate the supplements you are taking. You may choose to leave some in or switch some of them up. Please note, taking out the supplements WILL NOT cause you to gain weight. At this point, you will just be keeping them in for their health and wellness benefits.

In regards to water, because you are no longer looking to lose weight, you only need enough water to keep you hydrated.

STILL LOOKING TO LOSE??

For those of you still working towards your goal, later this week we will be talking about a game plan moving forward.

For now, continue with Personalizing the Plan and Maximizing your efforts and be sure to let us know if you have any questions.

PLEASE NOTE:

If you are done losing but want to join the next Group, I will be discussing the benefits of redoing the process to help solidify the weight you have lost and help the body level up in terms of health and wellness...when we discuss next steps later this week.

Please take time to head over to the Facebook Group and watch the quick video that accompanies this post.

CONTINUING TO LOSE OPTION 1 - REPEATING THE PROCESS

Let's Talk Option One Repeating the Process!

Repeating the Process means doing a complete reset of The Program and re-doing the Process over again week to week from the beginning.

Which is an effective option.

The idea being that you are restarting the process with your body now functioning at a more optimal level.

Don't overthink it, it's really just about approaching the second round (or 3rd, 4th, 5th) with Fresh Eyes, and being just as diligent and motivated as you were the first time around.

Keeping in mind each time you repeat the Process, it's key not to assume your body will respond in the same way because your body next time around will be functioning on a whole other level.

Some of you who have more weight to lose, may have to complete another few rounds to reach your goal. Have faith that each time your body will be working more and more in your favour, making the Process easier and easier.

The first time around, you will find yourself more focused on the physical elements of The Program what you are eating and how your body is responding.

You will find when you repeat the Process, it becomes more of a mental game. So, it is key to approach each new Group with Fresh Eyes.

If this was your first time through The Program and you are considering doing a reset, I would suggest reviewing the Fresh Eyes Post.

You will want to continue repeating the Process until you have reached your goal.

Some of you might reach your goal half way through the second round, or third or maybe even 4th or 5th round.

When you reach your goal, you can continue to follow through on the steps to help solidify your weight and finish The Program, OR start the Maintenance Phase.

You can redo The Program by signing up for the next Group Session or follow along on your own by utilizing the info from this current Group.

You can access any of the information, including all of the Posts, Videos and the Lives, through the Facebook Support Group for the next year.

It is suggested that you follow the days and weeks in order starting with Week 1 (Day 8). Anything that is not included in this Workbook, such as accompanying Videos, can be found in the Support Group by using the Guides.

Keep in mind, we will not be answering questions in the Group after it ends, but be sure to follow me over on my social media platforms and I will be going Live over on my public Facebook page the week leading up to the next Group to answer any questions.

If your plan is to continue with the next Group, you can continue to lose with Personalizing the Plan until it starts. Or, if you are feeling like the next few weeks are going to be chaotic or busy or you know you will be having a hard time staying focused, there is also the option of implementing Back on Track to bridge the gap.

Back on Track is best used when you go off the rails and indulge. But during stressful or chaotic times, if you feel like you don't have the capacity to focus on your food choices as much as you like in between groups, then BOT can be a good option.

My preference would be for you to continue Personalizing the Plan in preparation for doing a complete reset in the next Group.

For those of you who may be behind in the Group and following on your own timeline:

- Do your best to complete as many weeks as possible before repeating the Process.
- If you are doing The Program on your own, then be sure to complete the full 12 weeks before you start again.
- If your plan is to do the next Group, then keep following along as far as you can and then reset with the new Group.

Repeating the Process is an effective method to continue to lose for many reasons, as each time The Program works just as well, if not better. There is an advantage in knowing what's to come and how to step up your game and capitalize on the Process

It also gives the option for the body to level up your health and wellness as it challenges the body to address issues and continue to make change.

CONTINUING TO LOSE OPTION 2 - PERSONALIZING THE PLAN

Let's Talk Option 2 Personalizing the Plan.

"Personalizing The Plan" is doing all of the things, and making sure to maximize everything you need to do to help keep the body focused on fat loss to get the fat out.

This is the technique you have been using these last 2 weeks and also the method I used for my personal one on one clients. It is very effective.

When Personalizing The Plan, it is assumed you are looking to lose more weight, so you need to be as diligent and as consistent as possible and use all of the tools you have learned along the way to keep the scale moving.

Every minute of every day, you are being in tune to your body's needs to help it focus on, and get into detox and keep it in detox for as long as possible to help the body focus on fat loss.

When Personalizing The Plan, you can still implement Back on Track when you find yourself indulging or going off Plan.

Remember that PTP is checking in at every single meal and snack. It's making the best food choices based on the Guidelines. It's being super in tune to portions, and it's making sure to relentlessly Maximize.

Regardless of which method you choose, keep in mind the scale will still fluctuate and your hunger levels will continue to change day to day.

Be sure to review the Maximizing and the Hunger Posts and remember, although we won't be answering questions, all the information stays in the Facebook Group for you to access for the next year, should you need to review anything.

Being clear about next steps is key, as you don't want to find yourself flip flopping from one technique to another. Set your goal and be clear about your intention.

Continue to work hard and be relentless when it comes to finishing the Process and not only reaching your goal, but solidifying the weight that you have lost.

Personalizing The Plan is an effective method for reaching your goal, so continue to stay focused and visualize the end game. Think of Personalizing The Plan as following a diet specifically designed for you.

After these past few months, you know your body's needs more than anyone and after completing this Process, you are more in tune than ever. Your body is on your side and wants the fat gone just as much as you do.

The benefits of following your Personalized Plan over repeating the Process, is it gives you more flexibility in your day to day food choices.

BRIDGING THE GAP BETWEEN GROUPS

Let's talk bridging the gap between the end of this Group & repeating the Process again.

Repeating the Process is an effective way to lose. If that's your plan, I suggest you review the Fresh Eyes Post. It will give you some insight into things to keep in mind each time you repeat the Process.

If you are planning on doing a repeat of The Program on your own, it's a great idea to get a few weeks of Personalizing The Plan under your belt as you want to be as in tune to your body's needs as possible before you jump back into the week to week structure of a reset.

If you are planning on doing the next Group, I would ideally like to see you using the Personalizing The Plan technique until the start date.

If you do find yourself indulging/enjoying/partaking in the weeks in between groups, be sure to use Back on Track as often as you need and then continue on with Personalizing The Plan.

If you find you are at capacity and still want to lose, but know you won't have the same kind of time and energy to give to the Process on your own, you might want to consider using the Back on Track Method to bridge the gap.

Back on Track is ideally reserved for when you go off the rails, but given the added stress and chaos of this year, it could be exactly what you need to help calm the body and enable it to stay more focused on fat loss.

Remember that Personalizing the Plan can also look a lot like the original Food Plan with the added flexibility of skipping or switching up your snacks.

At the end of the day, it's all about intention and what feels best.

TO RECAP:

If you are done losing, you are going to follow the Maintenance Protocol. If you are looking to continue your journey, you are going to:

A: Re-do the program in the next Group

B: Re-do the program on your own using the info in this Group

C: Continue with Personalizing The Plan until you reach your goal and will use BOT for the times you indulge.

If you choose A or B, you are going to Bridge the Gap between this Group and the next by:

A: Personalizing The Plan using Back on Track when needed until you start the next Group

B: Sticking with the original Food Plan (BOT), and working the basics before starting The Program again.

ON A FINAL NOTE:

If you are behind in the Group and working through any of the previous weeks, continue to work at your own pace and be sure to reach out if you have any questions.

If you have signed up for the next Group, you can continue with moving forward from where you are at and then reset when the new Group starts.

LET'S REVISIT CELEBRATORY WEEKENDS

Keep in mind, you can be hard core about your journey and still enjoy those special moments in life on the way to reaching your goal. So, at the end of the day, it's more about how you want to feel afterwards.

Here my 5 top tips for staying on track:

1. **Take some time to set your intention before the weekend. Are you going to stay on plan, choose to indulge, or take each day as it comes?**

   There is no right or wrong answer to this, it's all about how you want to feel when it's time to get back at it.

2. **Regardless of what you plan to do, make a point of eating normally the day of any big event or in anticipation of a big/festive meal.**

   - Meaning, follow the Food Plan leading up, which will help keep your digestive system stimulated so going into the meal, you digest it better, and feel less bloated after eating a bigger meal.

3. **Eating all meals and snacks leading up will prevent you from overeating.**

   - Including starting your day with higher protein like eggs or full fat greek yogurt, even if you usually skip it.

4. **Starting your day higher in protein and fat and minimal carbs, for example eggs over oatmeal, will get your body working harder from the get-go and give you more sustaining energy.**

   - Also, if you have carbs like cereal, oatmeal or bread, you run more of a risk of setting yourself up to crave carbs and sugar all day and if there is lots of food around, you are going to be tempted by it if you are already craving it.

5. **Stay on top of your water and try to start earlier in the day.**

   - If you are on the road or out and about, make a plan and get it in when you can.

And finally, keep in mind:

At the end of the day, even if you eat your face off, you can't make a pound of fat in a day, overnight, or weekend...so all you need to do is get right back on track the next day.

END OF PROGRAM FAQS

With the program coming to an end, we have compiled a list of some of the most frequently asked questions.

1. **Will we have access to this group when it's done?**

   Yes! Although we stop posting and answering questions on Monday, April 11, you will still be able to access the group to review the information after we are done.

2. **Will the Spring/Summer Group have its own Support Group?**

   Yes, each new group has its own separate support group.

3. **Do I need to keep taking the supplements?**

   If you have reached your goal and you are ready for maintenance you can decide what you want to continue to take for health benefits. Otherwise, you don't need to keep taking them to maintain your weight.

   If you are still looking to lose you have options, you can take a break from the supplements between groups or keep taking them. There are benefits to both options so it's really personal preference.

   Same rules apply for the ACV or Lemon water

4. **I'm concerned about gaining weight in between groups. How do I avoid that?**

   Be sure to review the post on "How not to gain weight back"

   Be sure to have a plan and be clear on next steps, review the Next Steps Options Posts.

   Be sure to use BOT when you indulge to the point you feel off and or weight is up.

5. **How do I register for the next Group?**

   Sign Up Page on our website www.ginalivy.com

6. **Do I need Facebook to sign up for the new Group or can I just use the New App?**

   The App is to be used alongside the Facebook support group as a companion app.

   Our stand-alone app will be ready in Sept 2022 so you will need Facebook to follow until then

7. **Where do I download the App?**

   You can follow the directions sent by email at the time of purchase or download from the Apple App Store or Google Play Store.

8. **What if I didn't get a code for the New Group or App?**

Any administrative questions should be sent to through the website www.ginalivy.com or email weightloss@ginalivy.com as they have the resources to help

Any App specific questions can be directed to techsupport@ginalivy.com

9. **Is there a new PDF Booklet for the Spring/Summer Group?**

Yes! There will be a new updated version of the PDF Booklet available for the Spring/Summer Group

You can still use the Winter version and then print off any new info from the file section in the Facebook Group.

10. **What if I have feedback about the program I would like to share?**

We want to hear from you, so please fill out the Survey posted in the group and share your thoughts

11. **How do I find you in between groups?**

You can follow Gina over on her social media pages

Facebook: https://www.facebook.com/ginalivy

Instagram: https://instagram.com/ginalivy?utm_medium=copy_link

Gina will also be going Live on her public page 9am EST the week leading up to the Spring/Summer group.

WINTER 2022 GROUP: TRACKING SHEET

Use the chart below to track your progress throughout the Winter 2022 Group. This chart can be used to help you pick up on patterns of behaviors and responses and give you a better idea of what weight loss looks like specifically to you. Feel free to fill in all or none of the columns or personalize what types of things you want to track in the notes section. Happy tracking!

January 2022

| | | | \|Meals and Snacks\| | | | | | | | |
Date	Weight	Water	B	S1	L	S2	S3	D	Supplements	Notes (i.e., NSVs, BMs, Exercise, Sleep, Bonus snacks, etc.)
Jan 10			☐	☐	☐	☐	☐	☐	☐	
Jan 11			☐	☐	☐	☐	☐	☐	☐	
Jan 12			☐	☐	☐	☐	☐	☐	☐	
Jan 13			☐	☐	☐	☐	☐	☐	☐	
Jan 14			☐	☐	☐	☐	☐	☐	☐	
Jan 15			☐	☐	☐	☐	☐	☐	☐	
Jan 16			☐	☐	☐	☐	☐	☐	☐	
Jan 17			☐	☐	☐	☐	☐	☐	☐	
Jan 18			☐	☐	☐	☐	☐	☐	☐	
Jan 19			☐	☐	☐	☐	☐	☐	☐	
Jan 20			☐	☐	☐	☐	☐	☐	☐	
Jan 21			☐	☐	☐	☐	☐	☐	☐	
Jan 22			☐	☐	☐	☐	☐	☐	☐	

Date	Weight	Water	Meals and Snacks						Supplements	Notes (i.e., NSVs, BMs, Exercise, Sleep, Bonus snacks, etc.)
			B	S1	L	S2	S3	D		
Jan 23			☐	☐	☐	☐	☐	☐	☐	
Jan 24			☐	☐	☐	☐	☐	☐	☐	
Jan 25			☐	☐	☐	☐	☐	☐	☐	
Jan 26			☐	☐	☐	☐	☐	☐	☐	
Jan 27			☐	☐	☐	☐	☐	☐	☐	
Jan 28			☐	☐	☐	☐	☐	☐	☐	
Jan 29			☐	☐	☐	☐	☐	☐	☐	
Jan 30			☐	☐	☐	☐	☐	☐	☐	
Jan 31			☐	☐	☐	☐	☐	☐	☐	

January Notes:

_____

_____

_____

_____

_____

February 2022

Date	Weight	Water	B	S1	L	S2	S3	D	Supplements	Notes (BMs, Exercise, Period, Stress, Bonus snacks, etc.)
			Meals and Snacks							
Feb 1			☐	☐	☐	☐	☐	☐	☐	
Feb 2			☐	☐	☐	☐	☐	☐	☐	
Feb 3			☐	☐	☐	☐	☐	☐	☐	
Feb 4			☐	☐	☐	☐	☐	☐	☐	
Feb 5			☐	☐	☐	☐	☐	☐	☐	
Feb 6			☐	☐	☐	☐	☐	☐	☐	
Feb 7			☐	☐	☐	☐	☐	☐	☐	
Feb 8			☐	☐	☐	☐	☐	☐	☐	
Feb 9			☐	☐	☐	☐	☐	☐	☐	
Feb 10			☐	☐	☐	☐	☐	☐	☐	
Feb 11			☐	☐	☐	☐	☐	☐	☐	
Feb 12			☐	☐	☐	☐	☐	☐	☐	
Feb 13			☐	☐	☐	☐	☐	☐	☐	
Feb 14			☐	☐	☐	☐	☐	☐	☐	
Feb 15			☐	☐	☐	☐	☐	☐	☐	

Date	Weight	Water	Meals and Snacks						Supplements	Notes (i.e., NSVs, BMs, Exercise, Sleep, Bonus snacks, etc.)
			B	S1	L	S2	S3	D		
Feb 16			☐	☐	☐	☐	☐	☐	☐	
Feb 17			☐	☐	☐	☐	☐	☐	☐	
Feb 18			☐	☐	☐	☐	☐	☐	☐	
Feb 19			☐	☐	☐	☐	☐	☐	☐	
Feb 20			☐	☐	☐	☐	☐	☐	☐	
Feb 21			☐	☐	☐	☐	☐	☐	☐	
Feb 22			☐	☐	☐	☐	☐	☐	☐	
Feb 23			☐	☐	☐	☐	☐	☐	☐	
Feb 24			☐	☐	☐	☐	☐	☐	☐	
Feb 25			☐	☐	☐	☐	☐	☐	☐	
Feb 26			☐	☐	☐	☐	☐	☐	☐	
Feb 27			☐	☐	☐	☐	☐	☐	☐	
Feb 28			☐	☐	☐	☐	☐	☐	☐	

February Notes:

_____

_____

_____

_____

March 2022

Date	Weight	Water	B	S1	L	S2	S3	D	Supplements	Notes (i.e., NSVs, BMs, Exercise, Sleep, Bonus snacks, etc.)
			colspan-Meals and Snacks							
Mar 1			☐	☐	☐	☐	☐	☐	☐	
Mar 2			☐	☐	☐	☐	☐	☐	☐	
Mar 3			☐ ☐	☐ ☐	☐ ☐	☐ ☐	☐ ☐	☐ ☐	☐	
Mar 4			☐ ☐	☐ ☐	☐ ☐	☐ ☐	☐ ☐	☐ ☐	☐	
Mar 5			☐ ☐	☐ ☐	☐ ☐	☐ ☐	☐ ☐	☐ ☐	☐	
Mar 6			☐ ☐	☐ ☐	☐ ☐	☐ ☐	☐ ☐	☐ ☐	☐	
Mar 7			☐	☐	☐	☐	☐	☐	☐	
Mar 8			☐	☐	☐	☐	☐	☐	☐	
Mar 9			☐	☐	☐	☐	☐	☐	☐	
Mar 10			☐ ☐	☐ ☐	☐ ☐	☐ ☐	☐ ☐	☐ ☐	☐	
Mar 11			☐ ☐	☐ ☐	☐ ☐	☐ ☐	☐ ☐	☐ ☐	☐	
Mar 12			☐ ☐	☐ ☐	☐ ☐	☐ ☐	☐ ☐	☐ ☐	☐	
Mar 13			☐ ☐	☐ ☐	☐ ☐	☐ ☐	☐ ☐	☐ ☐	☐	
Mar 14			☐	☐	☐	☐		☐	☐	
Mar 15			☐	☐	☐	☐		☐	☐	

| Date | Weight | Water | Meals and Snacks | | | | | | Supplements | Notes (BMs, Exercise, Period, Stress, Bonus snacks, etc.) |
			B	S1	L	S2	S3	D		
Mar 16			☐	☐	☐	☐		☐	☐	
Mar 17			☐	☐	☐	☐		☐	☐	
Mar 18			☐	☐	☐	☐		☐	☐	
Mar 19			☐	☐	☐	☐		☐	☐	
Mar 20			☐	☐	☐	☐		☐	☐	
Mar 21			☐	☐	☐	☐		☐	☐	
Mar 22			☐	☐	☐	☐		☐	☐	
Mar 23			☐	☐	☐	☐		☐	☐	
Mar 24			☐	☐	☐	☐		☐	☐	
Mar 25			☐	☐	☐	☐		☐	☐	
Mar 26			☐	☐	☐	☐		☐	☐	
Mar 27			☐	☐	☐	☐		☐	☐	
Mar 28			☐	☐	☐	☐	☐	☐	☐	
Mar 29			☐	☐	☐	☐	☐	☐	☐	
Mar 30			☐	☐	☐	☐	☐	☐	☐	
Mar 31			☐	☐	☐	☐	☐	☐	☐	

March Notes:

_____

_____

_____

_____

_____

April 2022

Date	Weight	Water	Meals and Snacks						Supplements	Notes (i.e., NSVs, BMs, Exercise, Sleep, Bonus snacks, etc.)
			B	S1	L	S2	S3	D		
Apr 1			☐	☐	☐	☐	☐	☐	☐	
Apr 2			☐	☐	☐	☐	☐	☐	☐	
Apr 3			☐	☐	☐	☐	☐	☐	☐	
Apr 4			☐	☐	☐	☐	☐	☐	☐	
Apr 5			☐	☐	☐	☐	☐	☐	☐	
Apr 6			☐	☐	☐	☐	☐	☐	☐	
Apr 7			☐	☐	☐	☐	☐	☐	☐	
Apr 8			☐	☐	☐	☐	☐	☐	☐	
Apr 9			☐	☐	☐	☐	☐	☐	☐	
Apr 10			☐	☐	☐	☐	☐	☐	☐	
Apr 11			☐	☐	☐	☐	☐	☐	☐	
Apr 12			☐	☐	☐	☐	☐	☐	☐	
Apr 13			☐	☐	☐	☐	☐	☐	☐	
Apr 14			☐	☐	☐	☐	☐	☐	☐	
Apr 15			☐	☐	☐	☐	☐	☐	☐	
Apr 16			☐	☐	☐	☐	☐	☐	☐	

Apr 17			☐	☐	☐	☐	☐	☐	☐	
Apr 18			☐	☐	☐	☐	☐	☐	☐	
Apr 19			☐	☐	☐	☐	☐	☐	☐	
Apr 20			☐	☐	☐	☐	☐	☐	☐	
Apr 21			☐	☐	☐	☐	☐	☐	☐	
Apr 22			☐	☐	☐	☐	☐	☐	☐	
Apr 23			☐	☐	☐	☐	☐	☐	☐	
Apr 24			☐	☐	☐	☐	☐	☐	☐	

April Notes:

_____

_____

_____

_____

_____

Manufactured by Amazon.ca
Bolton, ON